Childhood Emergencies in the Office, Hospital, and Community: Organizing Systems of Care

Committee on Pediatric Emergency Medicine
American Academy of Pediatrics

James S. Seidel, MD, PhD, *Editor*
Jane F. Knapp, MD, *Editor*

American Academy of Pediatrics
141 Northwest Point Boulevard
Elk Grove Village, IL 60007

Second edition
First edition, 1992

Edition 1 of this manual was issued under the title: *Emergency Medical Services for Children: The Role of the Primary Care Provider*

Library of Congress Catalog No: 00-100184
ISBN: 1-58110-043-4
MA0052

Quantity prices on request. Address all inquiries to:
American Academy of Pediatrics
141 Northwest Point Boulevard, PO Box 927
Elk Grove Village, Illinois 60009-0927

The recommendations in this publication do not indicate an exclusive course of treatment or serve as a standard of medical care. Variations, taking into account individual circumstances, may be appropriate.

Cover photo courtesy of Captain Rick McClure, Los Angeles City Fire Department

Contents

Acknowledgments

The editors are indebted to the many authors and committee members who gave of their time and personal resources to write and review chapters for this manual. We would also like to thank Bill Wilkinson for his kindness in providing a wonderful environment in which to edit this book and Patty Zimmerman for her outstanding copy editing. In addition, we are indebted to Sue Tellez of the American Academy of Pediatrics, whose dedication and professionalism are an inspiration.

Contributors

Jean Athey, PhD
Former Program Director EMS-C
Health Resources and Services Administration
Maternal and Child Health Bureau
Rockville, MD

Jill Baren, MD, FACEP
Assistant Professor of Medicine and Pediatrics
University of Pennsylvania
  School of Medicine

Stephen Bickler, MD, FACS
Assistant Clinical Professor of Surgery
University of California at San Diego

Margaret Dolan, MD, FAAP
Assistant Professor of Pediatrics
Virginia Commonwealth University
  School of Medicine

Sharon Dorfman, ScM, CHES
President, SPECTRA
Ponce Inlet, FL

M. Denise Dowd, MD, MPH, FAAP
Associate Professor of Pediatrics
University of Missouri at Kansas City
  School of Medicine

Susan Fuchs, MD, FAAP, FACEP
Associate Professor of Pediatrics
Northwestern University
  School of Medicine

Michael Gerardi, MD, FAAP, FACEP
Director, Pediatric Emergency Medicine
Atlantic Health System
Morristown, NJ

Janis Guerney, Esq, Assistant Director
Department of Federal Affairs
American Academy of Pediatrics
Washington, DC

Deborah P. Henderson, PhD, RN
Assistant Professor of Pediatrics
University of California at Los Angeles
  School of Medicine

Dee Hodge III, MD, FAAP, FACEP
Associate Professor of Pediatrics
Washington University
  School of Medicine

Robert Kennedy, MD, FAAP
Associate Professor of Pediatrics
Washington University
  School of Medicine

Jane Knapp, MD, FAAP, FACEP
Professor of Pediatrics
University of Missouri at Kansas City
  School of Medicine

Stephan E. Lawton, Esq.
Hogan & Hartson
Washington, DC

Mary Letourneau, MD, FAAP, FACEP
Associate Professor of Pediatrics
University of California at Los Angeles
  School of Medicine

Jan Luhmann, MD
Instructor in Pediatrics
Washington University
  School of Medicine

Karin McCloskey, MD, FAAP
Assistant Professor of Pediatrics
University of Texas, Southwestern
  School of Medicine

Lee Pyles, MD, FAAP
Assistant Professor of Pediatrics
University of Minnesota
  School of Medicine

Mark Roback, MD, FAAP
Assistant Professor of Pediatrics
University of Colorado
  School of Medicine

Lance Rodewald, MD, MPH, FAAP
Centers for Disease Control and Prevention
Atlanta, GA

James Seidel, MD, PhD, FAAP
Professor of Pediatrics
University of California at Los Angeles
  School of Medicine

Joseph Simon, MD, FAAP
Medical Director
Scottish Rite Children's Hospital
Atlanta, GA

Deborah Mulligan-Smith, MD, FAAP, FACEP
Medical Director, Pediatric Services
  and Emergency Medical
  Services for Children
North Broward County Hospital District
Ft Lauderdale, FL

Vincent Tamariz, MD, FAAP
Instructor in Pediatrics
University of California at Los Angeles
  School of Medicine

Susan Tellez, Manager
Department of Committees and Sections
American Academy of Pediatrics
Elk Grove Village, IL

Robert Wiebe MD, FAAP, FACEP
Professor of Pediatrics
University of Texas
Southwestern Medical Center

George Woodward, MD, FAAP
Associate Professor of Pediatrics
University of Pennsylvania
  School of Medicine

Jean Wright, MD, MBA, FAAP
Professor of Pediatrics
Emory University
  School of Medicine

Timothy Yeh, MD, FAAP
Director, Critical Care
Children's Hospital Oakland
Oakland, CA

Amanda Vaughn
Summer Associate
Hogan & Hartson
Washington, DC

Preface

Emergency care is a critical component of the healthcare of children. Although pediatric emergency medicine is now a recognized subspecialty, most children present for emergency care in physicians offices, clinics, and community emergency departments. It is important for primary-care physicians to know how and when to access acute and critical services for their patients, the available facilities and resources in their communities, and how the "medical home" integrates within the emergency medical services system.

The intent of the first edition of the Committee on Pediatric Emergency Medicine (COPEM) manual, titled *Emergency Medical Services for Children: Role of the Primary Care Provider,* was to encourage each pediatrician, especially primary-care physicians, to participate in Emergency Medical Services for Children (EMS-C) in their communities. In addition, it introduced the concept of EMS-C as part of an integrated system of care that included an important component termed the "medical home." The challenge was to examine the emergency preparedness of the office and hospitals that care for critically ill and injured children.

This edition of the "Blue Book," titled *Childhood Emergencies in the Office, Hospital, and Community: Organizing Systems of Care,* reflects the maturation of the subspecialty and increased knowledge about the organization and practice of pediatric emergency and critical care medicine. In the 6 years since the publication of the earlier manual, many important changes have taken place in the provision of EMS-C. Every state and territory of the United States has received federal funding through the EMS-C program to develop and implement integrated systems of care. However, there is still great variability in the provision of high-quality pediatric emergency care and access to it throughout the United States and its territories. As a result, the American Academy of Pediatrics has fostered the organization of a Committee on Pediatric Emergency Medicine (COPEM) in all of its chapters. These committees are charged with improving services within their states and localities.

This book will help primary-care physicians examine the state of the art of pediatric emergency care nationally and provide them with a resource guide to examine the services in their own communities. Preparation takes place at many levels, and successful coordination of preparation leads to a "seamless" system of care that can improve outcomes. The book is divided into seven parts, summarized as follows:

- *Individual preparation* examines the role of the primary care physician and medical home in EMS-C; the preparation of parents, caretakers, and children for emergencies; and the need for psychological first aid.
- *Office preparation* concentrates on office policies, procedures, and general preparedness to manage acute emergencies.
- *Hospital preparation* examines the resources that should be in place in all community hospitals to adequately address the emergency-care needs of children.
- *Community preparation* addresses special situations, other emergency-care sites, geographical differences in care and resources, and advocacy concerns.
- *Transport preparation* deals with secondary transport from the office and between facilities.
- *Prevention preparation* stresses primary prevention in the three important areas of injury, immunization, and family violence.
- *EMS-C at the national level* describes the federal initiatives to improve pediatric emergency care.

An appendix provides an extensive updated list of available resources for information, patient care, advocacy, and education.

This book is the result of a collaborative effort by emergency physicians, pediatricians, and the AAP staff. Our intent has been to provide a reference manual that we hope you will use to improve pediatric emergency care in your community.

James Seidel, MD, PhD, FAAP,
Editor

Jane Knapp, MD, FAAP, FACEP,
Editor

Part I

Practitioner Preparation

Emergency Medical Services for Children (EMS-C) consists of a continuum of care from problem identification, through all phases of out-of-hospital and hospital care, to rehabilitation and community activ-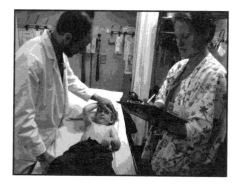ities. The individual commitment of office and hospital practitioners is key to the success of the system. Individual responsibilities include: preparing oneself for emergencies, injury and illness prevention, advocating EMS-C, and preparing children and their families to cope with emergencies. This part of the book presents materials on all of these important aspects.

Chapter 1

Role of the Primary-Care Physician in EMS-C

Key Roles for the Primary-Care Physician

1. Educator
2. Triage officer
3. Emergency-care physician
4. Consultant
5. Advocate
6. Disaster manager

Introduction

Preparation begins with the individual. It comprises the acquisition and maintenance of knowledge and the development of attitudes and skills that will facilitate the provision of care. Such preparation can be accomplished by continuing education, through specific training programs such as Pediatric Advanced Life Support (PALS), Advanced Pediatric Life Support: The Pediatric Emergency Medicine Course (APLS), Advanced or Basic Trauma Life Support (ATLS, BTLS), and by practice in preparing families and children to deal with emergencies.

Serving as the child's medical home, the primary-care physician is responsible for continuity of care. Figure 1 illustrates the central importance of that role and its relation to other components of the EMS system. This chapter defines the roles of the primary-care physician in EMS-C and the means for fulfilling these roles as educator, triage officer, emergency-care physician, consultant, child advocate, and participant in disaster management.

The Educator Role

The primary-care physician's most visible role is that of educator and the most important educational message is that of prevention. Effective prevention strategies include illness and intentional and unintentional injury prevention and access to poison control information (see Chapter 23).

The primary-care physician has the family's trust and therefore has a unique opportunity to have an effect on the knowledge, attitudes, and skills of family members. The physician should take advantage of this opportunity to educate families on

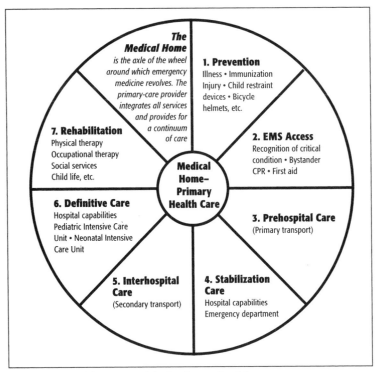

Fig 1. Medical home model of primary health care.

appropriate access to emergency care, seat-belt and bicycle helmet use, and the appropriate storage of alcohol and firearms.

The primary-care physician must educate the patient and parents in appropriate emergency response to illness or injury. Important questions to be addressed include:

- How do I decide whether to call the primary-care physician's office or to go directly to the emergency department?
- Which is the most appropriate hospital in the community for childhood emergencies?
- When should I drive to the emergency department rather than call for an ambulance?
- How do I access emergency care?
- What limitations does my insurance plan place on the location of the provision of emergency care?

See Chapter 3, "Preparing the Parent and Child to Cope with Emergencies," and Chapter 7, "Emergency Services and Managed Care," for more information.

Be aware of local school and child care policies with regard to the care of the acutely ill or injured child. See Chapter 19 for more information on emergencies at school.

Teach parents the importance of learning basic life support (BLS) and first aid through the American Heart Association (AHA), the American Red Cross, or their local hospital, fire department, or rescue squad. Lend your expertise as an instructor for BLS, first-aid, or PALS courses in your community. Make yourself available to organizations such as the PTA, schools, child care agencies, and so forth, for educational programs on child health.

Triage Officer

Be prepared to direct families to appropriate levels of emergency care in your community. To do so requires a working knowledge of the resources available in the community as well as how to appropriately access the emergency-care system.

Emergency-Care Physician

In spite of anticipatory guidance in regard to access to emergency care, children often present to the office with an emergency. Therefore, obtain and maintain your knowledge and skills in resuscitation and stabilization. This can be done through participation in PALS, APLS, and other resuscitation courses and in having practice mock codes in the office. Ensure that the office staff has BLS training and that the office is appropriately equipped for emergencies (see Chapter 5).

Consultation and Advocacy

Children are generally cared for in systems that were primarily designed for adults. Studies indicate that 90% of children requiring emergency care are treated not in a free-standing children's hospital emergency department, but rather in a general hospital, office, or urgent-care center. In a typical general hospital emergency department, from 25% to 33% of patients are children. Nationally, only 10% of ambulance responses are for pediatric patients; therefore, out-of-hospital care providers frequently not only are uncomfortable with the care of critically ill and injured children, but also lack the necessary skills for it. Most first-responding out-of-hospital providers have only BLS training and minimal exposure to pediatric emergency care. Their role in the EMS system positions them to provide care for children when they have little training and opportunity to maintain their pediatric care skills. The pediatrician can be a valuable consultant to out-of-hospital training programs, the emergency department, and other components of the EMS system that interact with pediatric patients.

Open lines of communication with emergency physicians in the community emergency department for notification of patients being referred to the emergency department and office follow-up of patients seen in the emergency department are important for continuity of care. This communication can be facilitated by application of modern technologies such as computers, fax machines, and e-mail to transfer information such as immunization status, drug allergies, and treatment records between various sites of care.

To advocate for EMS-C, pediatricians should:

- become knowledgeable about the types of equipment and supplies necessary for the provision of emergency care in the office and the emergency department.
- offer their services as consultants on matters of equipment, transport for critical care services, and requirements of children with special healthcare needs (see Chapters 5, 10, and 15).
- take part in the development of protocols for on- and off-line medical direction of their EMS systems as well as 911 dispatch protocols for pediatric emergencies.
- work with referral hospitals to ensure that interfacility transport and treatment protocols exist that will facilitate transfer of children requiring higher levels of care.
- participate in any mandatory or voluntary categorization of facilities process in their communities (see Chapter 20).
- help supplement out-of-hospital physician training for commonly occurring pediatric emergencies requiring transport. Such physicians should include 911 dispatchers, emergency medical technicians (EMTs), and paramedics.

- work with local and referral hospitals to ensure the existence of interfacility transport and treatment protocols that maximize local resources for the child.
- increase expertise on trauma resuscitation and care, and work with others in the community to ensure that appropriate trauma care is available within the EMS system.
- provide the link between the acute and the rehabilitation phases of care, ensuring the child optimal opportunity for the resumption of daily activities.

Disaster Management

Community disaster plans must address the needs of children in mass casualty situations. Recent EMS-C literature has focused on assisting primary-care physicians and emergency physicians in the planning for and management of disasters in which children are affected (see Chapter 16). Questions to be addressed include:

- What resources would have to be brought in and from where?
- What is the disaster plan of the area schools and child care facilities?
- Are the primary-care physicians integrated into the disaster plan?
- Is there an emergency telephone tree that could serve to alert the entire community?
- What is the local chapter of the American Academy of Pediatrics (AAP) doing to foster disaster management and education?

Summary

It takes committed participants to link all the components of EMS and EMS-C required for the provision of pediatric emergency care. This can be accomplished only by pediatricians working with emergency department and EMS personnel and law enforcement, fire department, school, and child care staff. This manual will enable you to become familiar with EMS-C issues and prepare you for your role in the prevention of illness and injury and the provision of pediatric emergency care. By increasing their knowledge, interest, and skills and by working with the community, pediatricians can make a difference in the development of systems of emergency care.

Suggested Reading

American Academy of Pediatrics Committee on Pediatric Emergency Medicine. The emergency physician and the office-based pediatrician: an EMSC team. *Pediatrics.* 1998;101:936–937

Dieckmann RA. *Pediatric Emergency Care Systems: Planning and Management.* Baltimore, MD: Williams & Wilkins; 1992

Durch JS, Lohr KN, eds. *Emergency Medical Services for Children.* Washington, DC: Institute of Medicine Division of Health Care Services, National Academy Press; 1993

Foltin G, Fuchs S. Advances in pediatric emergency medical service systems. *Emerg Med Clin North Am.* 1991;9:459–474

Haller JA, ed. *Emergency Medical Services for Children: Report of the 97th Ross Conference of Pediatric Research.* Columbus, OH: Ross Laboratories; 1989

Ludwig S, Selbst S. A child-oriented emergency medical services system. *Curr Probl Pediatr.* 1990;20:109–158

Seidel JS, Henderson DP, eds. *Emergency Medical Services for Children: A Report to the Nation.* Washington DC: National Center for Education in Maternal and Child Health; 1991

U.S. Department of Health and Human Services, Health Resources and Services Administration, Maternal and Child Health Bureau. *5 Year Plan: Emergency Medical Services for Children,* 1995–2000. Washington, DC: Emergency Medical Services for Children National Resource Center; 1995

Resources

You can make a difference in the lives of children and youth! Community Service Fact Sheet. EMSC National Resource Center, 1997, publication 602.

Training Programs for the Office Practitioner and Staff

Key Points in Training

1. The typical office sees a patient requiring emergency care weekly.

2. Morbidity and mortality of illness can be reduced with immediate and proper care.

3. Various-level training courses are available to update and maintain skills.

4. Mock codes provide essential experience in practicing skills and assessing facility preparedness.

Introduction

Life-threatening emergencies, which require immediate assessment and management of the resuscitation ABCs (airway, breathing, and circulation), are infrequent in the pediatric population compared with the adult population. However, the typical pediatric office is confronted with a patient requiring some form of emergency care at least once a week. Because morbidity and mortality of illness and injury can be reduced with immediate and proper care, all practitioners should be trained in the recognition and management of pediatric emergencies. The unpredictable nature and relative infrequency of these occurrences makes maintaining resuscitation skills a challenge.

A variety of formal training programs as well as informal exercises are available to office practitioners and their staffs for education in office preparedness for emergency situations. The initial step is participation in life-support courses.

Pediatric Basic Life Support (PBLS), Pediatric Advanced Life Support (PALS), Advanced Pediatric Life Support (APLS), and the Neonatal Resuscitation Program (NRP) offer information and training ranging from basic to advanced pediatric and neonatal life support.

The type of advanced educational course suited to an individual healthcare physician will depend on the scope of practice. All physicians, however, should know basic life support.

The Emergency Nursing Association (ENA) offers courses ranging from that for nurses with minimal exposure to significantly ill children (Emergency Nursing Pediatric Course) to more advanced courses designed to hone the skills of more experienced pediatric emergency nurses.

All of these courses provide information on pediatric resuscitation and must be updated or repeated every 2 years to maintain certification. Informal exercises such as mock codes may be periodically used to practice caring for pediatric emergencies. Additional reading materials are listed at the end of this chapter as another informal method of continuing education and practice in pediatric resuscitation.

Life-Support Courses

Adult basic and advanced life-support courses were developed in the 1960s. In 1988, resuscitation courses designed specifically for infants and children were introduced. The Pediatric Basic and Advanced Life-Support courses as well as the Neonatal Resuscitation Program offer resuscitation training unique to the pediatric population.

Pediatric Basic Life Support (PBLS)

The PBLS course is sponsored by the American Heart Association (AHA) and American Academy of Pediatrics (AAP) and is designed for lay persons interested in learning resuscitation techniques for infants and children. PBLS offers lay child-care providers an introduction to cardiopulmonary resuscitation (CPR) training and important information about injury prevention. The goal of this course is to reduce the number of childhood deaths caused by injuries or respiratory or cardiovascular problems. PBLS provides the foundation for training in pediatric advanced life support.

The Pediatric Basic Life Support Plus course and manuals also are available. PBLS Plus differs from PBLS by providing information about the use of barrier devices (mouth-to-mask) for use in CPR.

Information on the availability of PBLS courses may be obtained by contacting local chapters of the AHA or Red Cross. The national AHA telephone number is: (214) 373-6300. The national Red Cross number is: (202) 737-8300.

Basic Life Support for Healthcare Providers

Medical personnel can participate in the health providers' AHA Basic Life Support (BLS) course, which provides more advanced topics such as normal heart and lung anatomy and airway function and relief of airway obstruction.

Pediatric Advanced Life Support (PALS)

The AHA and AAP PALS course is targeted toward those who have completed a basic course and wish additional training in advanced life support of the pediatric patient. Current certification in basic or pediatric basic life support is a prerequisite.

The course focuses on recognition and management of impending or actual respiratory or cardiac failure. Topics covered include recognition of respiratory failure and shock, fluid therapy, use of emergency drugs, newborn resuscitation, and trauma. Skills stations offer further experience in basic life support and bag-valve-mask ventilation, advanced airway management, vascular access including intraosseous infusion, and cardiac rhythm disturbances. Pediatric resuscitation skills are actively learned and practiced through participation in case scenarios.

The emphasis of PALS is placed on the ABC (airway, breathing, and circulation) approach to pediatric resuscitation. The goal of this course is to prevent the progression of pediatric illness to cardiopulmonary arrest through early recognition and intervention.

Information regarding PALS courses provided in specific locations may be obtained by contacting the local affiliate of the AHA or a local CPR training center.

Advanced Pediatric Life Support (APLS): The Pediatric Emergency Medicine Course

APLS was developed through joint collaboration of the AAP and the American College of Emergency Physicians (ACEP). This course was developed for emergency physicians, general and subspecialist pediatricians, and family practitioners and nurses to increase their knowledge of pediatric emergency care. This course has recently been updated with the 1998 third edition of the manual.

The APLS course focuses on the acute management of common pediatric emergencies, both traumatic and medical. Topics covered include: respiratory distress, shock, cardiovascular disorders, trauma, environmental and toxicological emergencies, child abuse, altered level of consciousness, and status epilepticus. Additional sections provide information about advanced airway management including rapid sequence intubation (RSI), analgesia and sedation, use of medications, and an overview of emergency medical services for children. The manual also provides information on preparing for pediatric emergencies in the office and community hospital emergency departments.

The emphasis of the APLS course is placed on the initial 30-minute stabilization. The goal is to educate participants in the assessment and treatment of pediatric medical and surgical emergencies. The curriculum is geared toward the practitioner with more experience in advanced pediatric life support.

Information regarding attending or conducting an APLS course may be obtained by contacting AAP staff at 800/433-9016, ext 6795.

Neonatal Resuscitation Program (NRP)

The NRP is sponsored jointly by the AAP and AHA and is targeted at health professionals who take part in the delivery room resuscitation of the newborn infant. PBLS is recommended but not required.

The NRP course is designed to educate participants in a well-defined approach to the resuscitation of the newborn during the time immediately after birth. Topics covered in depth include: pathophysiology of asphyxia, initial steps in resuscitation, bag-mask ventilation, chest compressions, intubation, and appropriate usage of medication.

The emphasis of the NRP course is placed on preparation for the common emergencies associated with newborn deliveries. Case presentations and skills stations provide opportunity for participants to become familiar and comfortable with equipment required for newborn resuscitation. The goal of the course is to educate and train practitioners so that at least one person skilled in neonatal resuscitation may be in attendance at every delivery. The course can be tailored to the existing knowledge of the healthcare professionals participating so that, if basic skills have already been mastered, education can be directed to attaining more advanced knowledge and skills.

Information regarding NRP courses provided in specific locations may be obtained by contacting the AAP at (800) 433-9016, ext 6798.

Basic Trauma Life Support (BTLS)

The Basic Trauma Life Support (BTLS) course is provided through many local emergency agencies and academic centers. This course provides information on the basic procedures necessary for the stabilization and management of injured adults and children. It focuses on airway, breathing, circulation, disability prevention, exposure, and prevention of exsanguination. Information on BTLS may be obtained from Basic Trauma Life Support International Inc., 1 South, 280 Summit Avenue, Court B, Oakbrook Terrace, IL 60181, or by telephone: (800) 495-2857.

Advanced Trauma Life Support (ATLS)

The Advanced Trauma Life Support (ATLS) course is administered through the American College of Surgeons (ACS) and is targeted to emergency medicine and surgical personnel who care for injured patients. Although this course may not be helpful for the general practitioner, those interested in caring for injured children may benefit from the information and skills presented in this course. The curriculum includes initial assessment and stabilization of injured adults and children; advanced airway management including surgical airway procedures, vascular access, and chest tube placement; and anatomically focused assessment and management of various injuries. Information about ATLS may be obtained from the ACS Web site at www.facs.org.

Other Education Programs

Three programs are available through the National EMS-C Resource Alliance (NERA), 1124 West Carson Street, N-7, Torrance, CA 90502; (310) 328-0720. These programs may be helpful for training office staff in basic and advanced pediatric life support. They include:

1. The Intraosseous Infusion video and manual.
2. Basic Pediatric Airway Management, which includes an instructor's manual with case scenarios and a 16-minute full motion video on airway procedures. This program stresses recognition and management of respiratory distress and failure, use of airway adjuncts, and correct technique for bag-valve-mask ventilation.
3. Advanced Pediatric Airway Management, which includes a comprehensive instructor's manual, a complete slide set and instructor's script, a 28-minute full motion video on emergency airway procedures, and emergency airway scenarios. Skills include bag-valve-mask ventilation, endotracheal intubation, use of Magill forceps to remove airway foreign bodies, and delivery of endotracheal epinephrine.

Emergency Nursing Association Training Courses

The Emergency Nurses Association (ENA) provides courses and educational materials directed toward the emergency care of pediatric patients.

Emergency Nursing Pediatric Course (ENPC)

The ENPC is designed for nurses in emergency and general practice settings who may encounter pediatric patients requiring emergency care.

The course provides participants with knowledge of prevention strategies for injury and disease, as well as triage assessment and appropriate interventions for children requiring emergency care. Topics covered include: introduction to the pediatric patient, triage and initial assessment, respiratory failure and shock, and trauma and crisis intervention. Physician psychomotor skill stations provide additional experience in these topics as well as proper patient positioning, vascular access, fluids and medication administration, and pediatric resuscitation.

The emphasis of this course is to provide a nursing-based approach to prevention, assessment, and intervention for pediatric emergencies. The goals of the ENPC are to improve the care of the pediatric patient in the emergency-care setting and to increase the skill and confidence of emergency nurses who care for children.

Further information about ENA-sponsored products and the ENPC may be obtained by contacting the ENA at (800) 243-8362.

Nursing Assessment of Pediatric Emergencies

A self-learning text, *Nursing Assessment of Pediatric Emergencies,* can be used by nurses to improve their knowledge and skills in the assessment of pediatric patients. Nurses may obtain continuing education units from the ENA by completing the self-learning exercises in this book. The book is available through Springer Publishing.

Mock Codes

Life-support courses are the cornerstone of pediatric resuscitation education. These courses present a large body of information over a short period of time. To solidify the knowledge and skills learned in these courses, many pediatric clinics and offices, emergency departments, and hospitals have instituted mock code programs.

Pediatric mock codes are exercises in pediatric resuscitation, in which mannequins and programmed scenarios represent patients with pediatric emergencies. Participants are required to appropriately manage the emergency and "resuscitate the mannequin" as if it were a real clinical situation. Knowledge, attitudes, and skills obtained in the life-support courses are strengthened through repetition with the use of multiple different pediatric scenarios.

The mock code exercise emphasizes the ABCs of pediatric resuscitation learned in the life-support courses. This emphasis, with frequent repetition, is not readily available in most clinical settings. The goal of the exercise is to improve care of pediatric patients by keeping practitioners and staff current in the recognition and management of pediatric emergencies and well prepared to handle them in their clinical setting. (Sample mock codes are given in an Appendix to this chapter.)

Further information about instituting mock codes in any clinical setting may be obtained from the *Handbook of Pediatric Mock Codes* (see Suggested Reading at the end of this chapter). This handbook offers more than 35 different pediatric emergency scenarios and a step-by-step approach to pediatric resuscitation, education, and practice.

Summary

Training programs available to the office practitioner and staff provide education and practice in the emergency care of infants and children. These courses range from Basic Life Support appropriate for anyone interested in the care of pediatric patients to Advanced Pediatric Life Support directed toward experienced pediatric emergency-care physicians.

The greatest challenge is to maintain skills. This can be done through self-testing manuals and active practice resuscitations with the use of mock code exercises.

Poor outcomes for pediatric patients may be avoidable through prevention, early recognition, and immediate intervention. Maintaining a high level of preparedness through participation in the life-support courses and repeated practice by using mock code exercises is essential.

Suggested Reading

American Academy of Pediatrics, American Heart Association. *Pediatric Basic Life Support Plus.* Elk Grove Village, IL: American Academy of Pediatrics; Dallas, TX, American Heart Association; 1998

Bloom RS, Cropley C, eds. *Textbook of Neonatal Resuscitation.* Elk Grove Village, IL: American Academy of Pediatrics; Dallas, TX: American Heart Association; 1996

Chameides L, Hazinski MF, eds. *Pediatric Advanced Life Support.* Dallas, TX: American Heart Association; 1997

Haley K, Baker P, eds. *Emergency Nursing Pediatric Course: Provider Manual.* Park Ridge IL: Emergency Nurses Association; 1999

Hazinski MF, Chameides L, eds., American Academy of Pediatrics, American Heart Association, Subcommittee on Pediatric Resuscitation. *Pediatric Basic Life Support: Instructor's Manual.* Elk Grove Village, IL: American Academy of Pediatrics; Dallas, TX: American Heart Association; 1997

Henderson D, Brownstein D, eds. *Pediatric Emergency Nursing Manual.* New York, NY: Springer Publishing; 1994

Roback MG, Teach SJ, First LR, Fleisher GR, eds. *Handbook of Pediatric Mock Codes.* St. Louis, MO: Mosby Year Book; 1998

Strange GR, ed. *APLS Pediatric Emergency Medicine Course.* Elk Grove Village, IL: American Academy of Pediatrics; Dallas, TX: American College of Emergency Physicians; 1998

Resources

The *Advanced Pediatric Life Support* manual and *Textbook of Neonatal Resuscitation* are available for purchase from:

AAP Publications Department
141 Northwest Point Boulevard
PO Box 927
Elk Grove Village, IL 60009-0927
Telephone: (888) 227-1770

The *Emergency Nursing Pediatric Course: Provider Manual* and further information about pediatric nursing services may be obtained by contacting the ENA:

Emergency Nurses Association
216 Higgins Road
Park Ridge, IL 60068-5736
Telephone: (800) 243-8362

The American Heart Association has joined with the following four companies to be the sole distributors of emergency cardiovascular care material including *Pediatric Basic Life Support, Pediatric Basic Life Support Plus, and Pediatric Advanced Life Support* (textbook):

Channing L. Bete Co., Inc.
200 State Road
South Deerfield, MA 01373-0200
Telephone: (800) 611-6083
Fax: (800) 499-6464

LabSource, Inc.
319 West Ontario
Chicago, IL 60610-3606
Telephone: (800) 545-8823
Fax: (312) 944-7932

Laerdal Medical Corporation
167 Myers Corners Road
PO Box 1840
Wappingers Falls, NY 12590-8840
Telephone: (888) 562-4242
Fax: (800) 227-1143 or (914) 298-4545

Physio-Control
11811 Willows Road Northeast
PO Box 97006
Redmond, WA 98073-9706
Telephone: (800) 442-1142 (select option B)
Fax: (800) 426-8049

Appendix: Sample Mock Codes

Respiratory Distress: Pneumonia

Objectives:
1. Recognition of respiratory distress and impending respiratory failure.
2. Recognition of signs and symptoms of pneumonia.
3. Management of common complications of pneumonia.
4. Common etiologies and treatment of pneumonia.

History:
A 2-year-old boy with upper respiratory infection for 1 week presents with increased work of breathing, acute onset of fever, and increased cough.

Initial vital signs:
P 168, BP 102/70, RR 76.
If asked: temperature 40.1°C (R); estimated weight 15 kg.

Physical examination on arrival at ED:
General appearance: Pale, lying in mother's arms with nasal flaring and coughing, ill appearing.
If asked:
- HEENT: unremarkable except crusted nasal drainage.
  - Mucous membranes dry with 3 sec. capillary refill.
  - Neck: supple without meningeal signs.
  - CVR: tachycardic without murmur, femoral pulses palpated and slightly diminished.
  - Chest: using accessory muscles with intercostal, subcostal, and suprasternal retractions, fair aeration on right with diminished aeration in left base, crackles and bronchial

breath sounds in left middle and upper lobes, no wheezing auscultated.
- Abdomen: soft, nontender, no hepatosplenomegaly, bowel sounds diminished.
- Neuro: alert, looking around, nonfocal, anxious.

Further history given on request:
Patient has been drinking very little and not eating. He has complained of abdominal pain, and he has coughed up green-yellow mucous.

Expected interventions:	Complications:
1. 100% oxygen by face mask	• No improvement with oxygen
2. Monitors and pulse oximetry	• Pulse oximeter not reading
3. IV access attempt	• IV access attempt unsuccessful
4. Rapid glucose	
5. Call for CXR	
6. Antipyretics (PR acetaminophen)	

Repeat vital signs:
Pulse 178, BP 100/70, RR 63, temperature 39.2°C.

Labs:
Rapid glucose 89, ABG 7.18/70/86/-10 on 10L non-rebreather mask.

Progression:
The patient's respiratory rate slows to 12, pulse is 110, and he becomes unresponsive. Capillary refill 4–5 sec. Minimal breath sounds on the left.

Expected interventions:	Complications:
1. BVM assist breathing	• Copious secretions, vomiting
2. IO placement 20 cc/kg NS	
3. NG tube	• Suction not hooked to wall

Progression:
Perfusion remains poor.

Expected interventions: **Complications:**
1. Repeat 20 cc/kg NS bolus
2. IO antibiotics

Disposition:
Call 911 for transfer to hospital.

Discussion of objectives:

1. Recognition of respiratory distress and impending respiratory failure.

Respiratory distress is evidenced by abnormal respirations such as tachypnea, bradypnea, apnea, or increased work of breathing. Use of accessory muscles, nasal flaring, grunting, cyanosis, decreased mental status, and decreased air movement on auscultation are additional signs of respiratory distress found on physical examination.

The signs and symptoms of respiratory distress are useful for assessing the severity of illness and dictating the urgency of evaluation and therapy. The diagnosis is aided by obtaining an oxygen saturation by pulse oximetry.

Oxygen therapy and cardiac monitoring should be initiated immediately for patients in respiratory distress.

2. Recognition of signs and symptoms of pneumonia.

Pneumonia is an acute infection of the lung parenchyma, and classic signs include fever, cough, rales, and evidence of pulmonary consolidation on physical examination. Most care physicians also require radiographic evidence at some time in the course of the illness to corroborate the physical findings. However, roentgenogram changes can lag behind the clinical presentation initially as well as during recovery.

3. Management of common complications of pneumonia.

Common complications of pneumonia include copious secretions, bronchospasms and wheezing, hypoxia and hypercapnia, pleural effusion, empyema, and septic shock. Office support includes 100% oxygen, suctioning, nebulized beta-2 agonists, and vigorous support of perfusion with isotonic fluids.

Seizure Disorder: Status Epilepticus

Objectives:
1. Recognition of the patient in status epilepticus.
2. Differentiation of the possible etiologies of status epilepticus.
3. Identification of the key management strategies in status epilepticus.

Brief presenting history:
A 4-year-old boy with cerebral palsy, developmental delay, and a seizure disorder starts to have a generalized tonic-clonic seizure in the waiting room.

Initial vital signs:
HR 160, RR 28, BP 88/50.
If asked: temperature 38.5°C (R); estimated weight 12 kg (smaller than expected for age owing to chronic disease).

Initial physical examination:
General appearance: Generalized tonic-clonic seizure activity, eyes rolled back, gurgling breath sounds, pale skin color, copious oral secretions.

If asked:
- No focal neurologic findings, no signs of trauma.
  - Coarse breath sounds bilaterally.
  - Capillary refill time 3 sec.
  - Seizure affects all extremities, eyes deviated to the left.

Further history given on request:
PMHx: The patient was diagnosed with epilepsy at 6 months of age. He has been on **carbamazepine** and **valproic acid** since that time. His last seizure was 2 weeks ago with a usual frequency of one every few months lasting from 3 to 5 min. He has missed his last two appointments, and no recent anticonvulsant levels are known.

He has had upper respiratory symptoms for the past 3 days with low-grade fevers.

No known drug allergies, taking no other medications, no known ingestions.

There is no history of trauma. Prior to the seizure, he had been acting normally.

Expected interventions:
1. Assess ABCs.
2. 100% oxygen, suction the oropharynx.
3. Cardiac monitor, pulse oximeter.
4. Establish IV access NS 20 cc/kg IV/IO
5. **Lorazepam** 0.05–0.1 mg/kg IV/IO or **diazepam** 0.5 mg/kg PR

Complications:
- Airway compromise

- IV access unsuccessful requiring per rectal meds or IO placement

Repeat vital signs:
HR 175, RR 20, BP 80/45.

Labs:
Rapid glucose 178.

Progression:
Patient continues to have seizure; now 15 min in length.

Expected interventions:
1. Establish IV or IO access
2. **Lorazepam** 0.1 mg/kg IV/IO
3. Load with **phenytoin** 15–20 mg/kg IV/IO* (not to exceed 1 mg/kg/min) or **phenobarbital** 10–20 mg/kg IV/IO

Complications:
- Persistent seizure activity
- Rapid phenytoin load leads to cardiovascular collapse
- If phenobarbital used, patient becomes apneic

*__Fosphenytoin__ can now be given over 5 min without hemodynamic compromise.

Disposition:
Call 911 and transfer to hospital.

Discussion of Objectives:

1. Recognition of the patient in status epilepticus.
Status epilepticus is defined as continuous seizure activity for at least 30 min or as repeated seizures in which the patient does not return to baseline mental status.
Conscious or unconscious.
Morbidity can be significant with status epilepticus, including anoxia, hyperthermia, aspiration, metabolic acidosis, rhabdomyolysis, renal failure, and neurologic damage. Mortality ranges from 4% to 30% with recent decreases secondary to improved supportive care and pharmacotherapy.

2. Differentiation of the possible etiologies of status epilepticus.
The challenge of treating status epilepticus is to simultaneously stabilize the patient, direct therapy, and conduct a diagnostic evaluation to uncover the etiology of the status epilepticus.

3. Identification of the key management strategies in treating status epilepticus.
Management of status epilepticus is based on two principles:
(a) Maintain the patient's ABCs.
An oral or nasopharyngeal airway may be helpful in supporting the airway, and suction may be required to prevent aspiration of mucus and saliva. Oxygen is administered to prevent hypoxic injury. BVM-assisted respirations may be needed and, in extreme cases or if respiratory suppression occurs secondary to administration of anticonvulsants, endotracheal intubation may be required.
Hypotension may be secondary to an underlying process such as dehydration or may develop with prolonged seizure activity and requires isotonic fluid replacement. Occasionally, as in patients with septic shock, inotropic support may be required.
Hyperthermia may result from prolonged status epilepticus and must be addressed aggressively with antipyretics and external cooling measures such as cooling blankets.
During status epilepticus, it is important to secure patients from injury induced by the violence of convulsions. Posi-

tion patients on their sides (to maintain a patent airway) on a soft surface to protect their heads from banging.

(b) Be familiar with the pharmacologic options to stop convulsions and prevent further convulsions.

Benzodiazepines remain the initial drug of choice. **Lorazepam** 0.05–0.1 mg/kg provides a longer duration of action than **diazepam** or **midazolam**. **Diazepam** may be given rectally, 0.2–0.5 mg/kg. **Phenytoin** is the preferred second drug of choice because of the reduced respiratory depression and sedation compared with **phenobarbital**. The recent approval of **fosphenytoin** allows for a significantly more rapid administration without the serious cardiovascular side effects. **Fosphenytoin** is dosed in phenytoin equivalents (PE). Loading dose for emergent use is 15–20 mg/kg (PE) IV.

Shock: Sepsis

Objectives:
1. Recognition of the presentation of septic shock.
2. Management of relative hypovolemia.
3. Recognition and management of acidosis, hypoglycemia, and respiratory insufficiency.

Brief presenting history:
A 1-month-old infant in father's arms with a chief complaint of lethargy and poor feeding.

Initial vital signs:
P 200, BP 60/30, RR 60.
If asked: temperature 38.1°C; estimated weight 4.0 kg.

Physical examination on arrival to ED:
General appearance: Pale, gray, mottled, limp.
If asked:
- Eyes closed, minimally responsive to painful stimuli.
  - PERRL, AF flat, no retinal hemorrhages.
  - Breath sounds full and clear symmetrically without wheeze.
  - Heart tones remarkable for tachycardia only.
  - Capillary refill 4–5 sec, pulse weak.

- Abdomen nondistended, BS hypoactive, soft without mass.
- No external signs of trauma.

Further history given on request:
Child failed to wake for feeding as expected. Parents unable to arouse him. Refuses to take the breast. No history of ingestion or trauma. No urine output for more than 12 hours. Full term, NSVD, uncomplicated pregnancy, labor, and delivery. No medications.

Expected interventions:	**Complications:**
1. 100% oxygen by face mask (proper fit)	
2. Monitors: ECG and oximeter	
3. IV access attempts	• Unable to start IV
• IO placement	
4. NS bolus 20 cc/kg IO	
5. Labs: R-gluc	

6. Antibiotics:
   ceftriaxone 100 mg/kg IO
   and **ampicillin** 100 mg/kg IO	

Initial labs:
Rapid glucose 20.

Repeat vital signs:
P 60, BP not obtainable, RR 10.
ECG monitor, bradycardia; oximeter, not functioning.

Progression:
Mottled color becoming blue, agonal respirations, no response to needle sticks.

Expected interventions:	**Complications:**
1. Bag-valve-mask with 100% O_2	• No respiratory effort

2. Second 20 cc/kg NS bolus,
   followed by $D_{25}W$ infusion
   4 cc/kg (1 g/kg)

Repeat vital signs:
After preceding resuscitation: P 190, BP 75/35, perfusion improved slightly.

Disposition:
Call 911 for transfer to hospital.

Discussion of Objectives:

1. *Recognition of presentation of septic shock.*
   Septic shock is a syndrome of inadequate organ perfusion, requiring oxygen, intravascular fluid resuscitation, and antibiotics. Symptoms of shock evident in this patient include history of decreased activity, poor PO intake, and decreased urine output. Signs of shock are tachycardia, poor perfusion with cyanosis, prolonged capillary refill time, mottled skin, and altered mental status. Hypotension as displayed by low blood pressure is a *late* finding of shock in pediatrics and is indicative of impending cardiovascular collapse.

2. *Management of relative hypovolemia and poor cardiac output.*
   Isotonic crystalloid solution is administered initially as an IV bolus, 20 cc/kg, over a short (< 15 min) period of time. If reassessment of the patient's condition reveals persistent poor perfusion, the 20cc/kg bolus is repeated.

3. *Management of metabolic derangements including hypoglycemia and acidosis.*
   Glucose should be administered either as $D_{10}W$ at 10 cc/kg or $D_{25}W$ at 2–4 cc/kg to deliver approximately 0.5–1.0 g/kg of **dextrose.**

(Note: Mock codes are modified with permission from *Handbook of Pediatric Mock Codes,* MG Roback, SJ Teach, LR First, and GR Fleisher, eds. St Louis, MO: Mosby Year Book; 1998.)

Preparing the Parent and Child to Cope With Emergencies

Key Points in Parental Education on Emergencies

1. Pediatricians have a primary role in education of parents on prevention and appropriate response in an emergency.
2. Education can be accomplished in many ways and performed by other members of the primary-care team.
3. Parents need to assess the safety of their child at other caretaker sites.

Introduction

In a busy primary-care practice, it is difficult to find the time to educate parents and caregivers while providing quality clinical care of children. However, the statistics on preventable deaths and injuries in children provide a compelling reason to make parental education a priority. When parents and caregivers visit the office, the focus is on the health and well-being of their children, which makes every encounter a "teachable moment."

Information provided to parents according to a systematic plan, at age-appropriate intervals and utilizing other members of the primary-care team, can educate parents well. This plan can be supplemented by reading materials and posters or videos in waiting areas.

Educating Parents About Emergencies and EMS-C

The primary-care physician and office staff must be familiar with local EMS-C capability and organization. This can be a challenge, however, because many primary-care physicians serve a large geographic area with diverse EMS-C capabilities. In addition, many systems are still undergoing development and evolution.

Every community is different, varying with respect to 911 access, availability and accessibility of emergency and trauma care, number of pediatric referral care centers, and the sophistication of the EMS-C component of the EMS system. Primary-care physicians must have current information concerning changes that occur in the EMS-C component of the EMS system.

Parents usually have less knowledge than the pediatrician regarding a community's capabilities in EMS-C. Therefore, an important role for pediatricians is to teach parents about the emergency care available in their community. Pediatricians can obtain and use the AAP speaker's kit titled *Emergency Services for Children: A Child's Life Depends On It* for educating and raising awareness about EMS-C.

Several resources are available to aid the physician in the education of parents on pediatric emergencies. The Health Resources and Services Administration (HRSA) and the National Highway Traffic Safety Administration (NHTSA) publish a handbook for parents and people who care for children titled *How to Prevent and Handle Childhood Emergencies*. This handbook contains sections on how to get help for a sick or injured child and what to do until help arrives, as well as an emergency reference tape for parents and an extensive resource section. For information on obtaining copies of this handbook, contact the National EMS-C Resource Center at (703) 902-1203 and ask for product number 0576. The AAP also has a fact sheet available called *When Your Child Needs Emergency Medical Services*. Information on AAP educational materials may be found on the Web site at http://www.aap.org.

The physician can also prepare a practice-specific fact sheet for parents to use in case of an emergency (see Table 1). Make sure that written information is at a low literacy level by using simple one- or two-syllable words and, wherever possible, pictures and diagrams to clarify or reinforce educational messages. It is desirable to have materials available in Spanish and other languages encountered in one's practice. Provide references for parents and caregivers (books, videotapes, Internet sites, and so forth) where they can read and learn more about emergency care. Some of these references are listed at the end of this chapter. The EMS-C Web site (http://www.ems-c.org/family/Emerg10.html) has a page called *Knowing These Ten Things Could Save Your Child's Life* (see Table 2).

The AAP and the American College of Emergency Physicians (ACEP) recommend that parents and caregivers call 911 or their

Table 1.

Sample EMS-C Resource Sheet For Parents

• Regular office hours of the primary-care physician and the types of urgent problems that can be handled within the practice.
• The number to call at times other than regular office hours for urgent problems that would otherwise be handled within the practice.
• The name, address, and telephone number of the hospital emergency departments that the primary-care physician prefers. It is important for parents and caregivers to understand that the out-of-hospital providers will evaluate the situation and may determine that another facility can best provide the kind of care the child needs.
• The poison control number to call and the types of urgent problems best handled by poison control.
• The number to call first, even during regular office hours, when immediate EMS-C response is needed, and the types of emergencies in this category.

local emergency number whenever one or more of the following conditions arises:

• A child's condition becomes life threatening.
• The child is too unstable to be transported to the hospital by private means.
• Moving the child could cause further injury.
• A child needs the skills or equipment of paramedics or emergency medical technicians (EMTs).
• Rapid transport is necessary to prevent further injury or death.

It is further recommended that, when parents are not sure about what to do, they should make the call for help. NHTSA has developed a teaching curriculum titled "Make the Right Call" to help educate communities on how to access emergency care. It is available through NHTSA by calling (800) 424-9393 or accessing http://www.nhtsa.dot.gov on the Internet.

Encourage parents and caregivers to have a first-aid kit readily available. The kit should include items such as: a list of local

---

Table 2.

Knowing These Ten Things Could Save Your Child's Life

....

1. Know how to spot an emergency situation. An emergency situation exists if you think your child could die or suffer permanent harm unless prompt care is received.
2. Know how to contact your local emergency service. Use P.L.A.N. (**P**ost **L**ists of **A**ll Emergency **N**umbers) on or near every telephone as a guide.
3. Learn CPR and choking rescue procedures for infants and children.
4. Learn the basics of first aid. Knowing how to stop the bleeding from an open wound, manage shock, handle fractures, and control a fever could provide your child with the right amount of help in an emergency. Learning first aid will help you recognize an emergency.
5. Immunize.
6. Remember what to do if your child is in a car crash.
7. Understand what to do if your child is poisoned.
8. Learn what to do in case your child has a serious fall.
9. Know how to treat your child in case of a burn; that is, how to stop the process.
10. Be prepared on how to act in case your child has a seizure.

....

emergency phone numbers; hydrogen peroxide; antibiotic ointment; ibuprofen; calamine lotion; acetaminophen; cotton-tipped applicators; ready-to-use cold packs; a sling; adhesive strips; gauze; bandage rolls, bandage tape; cups or spoons to measure medications; syrup of ipecac and activated charcoal; scissors, sterile cotton balls; tweezers; antiseptic wipes; and elastic bandages. If a child has severe reactions to insect stings or certain foods, an EpiPen should be readily available.

Managed care organizations or other third-party payers that cover only designated physicians and facilities insure many families. Furthermore, there are notification rules affecting payment for emergencies and follow-up treatment. Encourage families to find out whether, when, and how to inform their insurers in case of a medical emergency. A brochure is available from the National EMS-C Resource Center called *When Your Child Needs Help in a Hurry.* This brochure gives parents advice about selecting and evaluating a healthcare plan based on considerations such as access to emergency care (see Chapter 7).

Sometimes children are brought directly to the primary-care physician's office for emergency care. It is important to establish clear, simple policies and procedures for office emergency management and referrals for emergency care. It is equally important to train everyone in the office who interacts with parents, caregivers, and children to conduct telephone and waiting-room screening for emergencies and to act quickly and appropriately in an emergency (see Chapter 2).

Because many children spend considerable time away from their homes and parents, it is important that other caregivers—teachers, day-care staff and sitters, relatives and neighbors, youth group leaders—know what to do in case of an emergency. It is the responsibility of the physician, parent, or guardian to ensure that these out-of-home settings are child-safe and that the caregivers have the information, resources, and skills necessary in an emergency situation. Urge parents and guardians to assess the safety of the environments in which their children spend time and to ensure the prevention awareness and emergency readiness of their children's part-time caregivers.

Educating Parents to Prevent Emergencies

Prevention is a basic component of EMS-C. Educating parents in the prevention of illness and injury is a high priority. The key in anticipatory guidance counseling is to convince parents that, although the risks are real, they can take measures to protect children from harm and to teach children safety. These measures include both indoor and outdoor child-proofing, protective behavior that adults should practice correctly and consistently to keep children safe, and safety habits to teach children when they are developmentally ready. Young people who are safety conscious and trained to act appropriately in an emergency situation may be able to save a life when another child needs help. Their ability to respond quickly and appropriately may be particularly crucial when an adult is not present, such as in latchkey situations. For more information on injury prevention, see Chapter 23. For available resources on injury prevention, consult the Resources section at the end of this chapter.

Summary

The pediatrician is the best person to teach prevention and educate the family on how to act in an emergency. Incorporating the following action points will ensure that this important education is accomplished.

1. Know your local EMS-C system and EMS-C components.
2. Contact your AAP chapter's Committee on Pediatric Emergency Medicine (COPEM) to learn more about EMS-C activities.
3. Inform parents and caregivers about when to call your office, when to seek emergency services, and when to contact poison control.
4. Make sure that your staff is trained and your office is equipped to respond quickly and appropriately to emergency calls and visits.
5. Provide age-appropriate injury prevention information to parents, caregivers, and children.
6. Teach parents, caregivers, and children who are old enough how to recognize and respond to pediatric emergencies.
7. Make materials on educational topics available to parents and caregivers.
8. Support the provision of community-based educational programs on preventing injuries to children and on handling emergencies.
9. Encourage parents and caregivers to take injury prevention and basic first aid, cardiopulmonary resuscitation (CPR), and other related classes.
10. Advocate for an effective EMS-C component within the existing system in the community.
11. Urge parents and caregivers to become advocates for EMS-C.

Suggested Reading

Christensen DW, Jansen P, Perkin RM. Outcome and acute care hospital costs after warm water near drowning in children. *Pediatrics.* 1997;99:715–721

Cohen LR, Runyan CW, Downs SM, Bowling JM. Pediatric injury prevention counseling priorities. *Pediatrics.* 1997;99:704–710

Ellis AA, Trent RB. Swimming pool drownings and near-drownings among California preschoolers. *Public Health Rep.* 1997;112:73–77

Gabrielli A, Layon AJ. Drowning and near drowning. *J Fla Med Assoc.* 1997;84:452–457

Gielen AC, McDonald EM, Forrest CB, Harvilchuck JD, Wissow L. Injury prevention counseling in an urban pediatric clinic: analysis of audiotaped visits. *Arch Pediatr Adolesc Med.* 1997;151:146–151

Hazinski MF, Francescuitti LH, Lapidus GD, Micik S, Rivara FP. Pediatric injury prevention. *Ann Emerg Med.* 1993;22:456–467

Knapp J. A call to action: the Institute of Medicine report on emergency medical services for children. *Pediatrics.* 1995;96:173–174

Mulligan-Smith, DA, ed. *How to Prevent and Handle Childhood Emergencies: A Handbook for Parents and People Who Care for Children.* U.S. Department of Health and Human Services, Health and Resources Services Administration, Maternal and Child Health Bureau. Washington, DC: Emergency Medical Services for Children National Resource Center; 1997

Nixon J, Pearn J, Wilkey I, Corcoran A. Fifteen years of child drowning: a 1967–1981 analysis of all fatal cases from the Brisbane Drowning Study and an 11 year study of consecutive near-drowning cases. *Accid Anal Prev.* 1986;18:199–203

Weinreich NK. Research in the social marketing process. The Social Marketing Place Web site, Weinreich Communications; 1996. http://www.social-marketing.com/process.html

Zuckerman BS, Parker S. Teachable moments: assessment as intervention. *Contemp Pediatr.* 1997;14:41–53

Resources

American Academy of Pediatrics Committee on Pediatric Emergency Medicine. Emergency Medical Services for Children: A Child's Life Depends on It. Speaker's Kit. Elk Grove Village IL: American Academy of Pediatrics; 1997

American Academy of Pediatrics Committee on Injury and Poison Prevention, Widome M, ed. *Injury Prevention and Control for Children and Youth.* 3rd ed. Elk Grove Village, IL: American Academy of Pediatrics; 1997

American Academy of Pediatrics Committee on Injury and Poison Prevention. The Injury Prevention Program (TIPP). Elk Grove Village, IL: American Academy of Pediatrics; 1994

American Academy of Pediatrics. Choking Prevention and First Aid for Infants and Children: Guidelines for Parents. Elk Grove Village, IL: American Academy of Pediatrics; 1999

Related AAP Policy Statements and Publication Dates

1. Access to Emergency Medical Care, 10/92
2. Consensus Report for Regionalization of Services for Critically Ill or Injured Children, 1/00
3. Consent for Medical Services for Children and Adolescents, 8/93
4. Death of a Child in the Emergency Department, 5/94
5. Guidelines for Pediatric Emergency Care Facilities, 9/95
6. Recommendations for Freestanding Urgent Care Facilities, 5/99
7. The Pediatrician's Role in Advocating Life Support Courses for Parents, 7/94
8. The Pediatrician's Role in Disaster Preparedness, 1/97
9. The Role of the Pediatrician in Rural EMSC, 5/98
10. The Use of Physical Restraint Interventions for Children and Adolescents in the Acute Care Setting, 3/97

Chapter 4

Psychological First Aid for Children Who Witness Violence

Key Points on Children Who Witness Violence

1. 3.3 million children witness violence each year.

2. Children who witness violence suffer problems similar to those of children who are physically abused.

3. Pediatricians have a role in the identification and referral of children who witness violence.

Introduction

A special concern in EMS-C is the care of children who have experienced or witnessed violence. Violence, in the form of homicide, suicide, assault and child abuse, is a threat to children's physical and emotional well being. It is common for children who have been physically injured secondary to violence to present for emergency services. It is much less common for the estimated 3.3 million children who witness domestic violence each year to receive prompt medical evaluation and mental health services. Yet, the available research finds that children who witness violence have risks for long-term consequences similar to those who experience physical injury. The concerns are more serious for those children who are repeatedly exposed to violence because they are additionally hampered in their efforts at recovery. The American Academy of Pediatrics (AAP) has prepared a resource fact sheet for pediatricians called "Some Things You Should Know about Witnessing Violence" that is available on its Web site (http://www.aap.org/advocacy/childhealthmonth/witness.htm).

Posttraumatic Stress Disorder

Posttraumatic stress disorder (PTSD) is a well-documented problem for children who witness or experience abuse and violence. The number and type of PTSD symptoms most often correspond to a child's level of exposure to the violence. To identify and care for these children, EMS-C must extend beyond the walls of the emergency department to the practice of the primary-care physician and to the provision of specialized mental health services.

Two processes are important to the care of the child who has witnessed violence. The pediatrician must be prepared through education and training for both. The first is *identification* and *screening*. Clinical experience with adults with PTSD suggests that early intervention produces the optimal result. Unfortunately, it is commonly found that children exposed to even extreme acts of violence do not receive timely psychological care. This information has prompted recommendations that pediatricians inquire about exposure to violence from both the child and the parents in the course of routine well-child visits. Child self-report is critical to successful screening because parents can deny or be poor observers of their child's traumatic reactions—especially in the acute phase. Later, parental report can help identify changes in behavior and the appearance of symptoms consistent with PTSD (Table 3). Children of battered women who are exposed to repeated family violence can be particularly disturbed and should be carefully screened. Positive responses necessitate a plan for intervention.

The second important process is *intervention*. Mental-health referrals are indicated for children who witness significant acts of violence or who have problems that can be related to witnessing violence. Yet, specialized mental-health services are frequently lacking. Here, the pediatrician has an additional role as

Table 3.

Symptoms of Posttraumatic Stress Disorder
••

Somatic complaints such as headache, stomachache, nausea, and vomiting	Moodiness
	Has obsessions
Anxiousness	Is withdrawn
Guilt	Is argumentative
Clinginess	Nervousness
Secretiveness	Feels persecuted
Sadness	Nightmares and
Inability to concentrate	sleeping difficulties
Irritability	Irrational fears

••

advocate for the development and acquisition of these kinds of services for the community. Specialized techniques are required because children may not respond to traditional methods of direct inquiry about the event or be able to verbalize their child-specific issues. Although not universally available, intervention models include combinations of art therapy, play therapy, story telling, group discussion or critical incident stress debriefing (CISD), and victim interview. Interventions can also take place in the classroom when an entire group of school children has been affected. It is important for the pediatrician to know the availability of community mental-health services and resources.

Many models for intervention and treatment for children who witness violence exist. The "witnesses to violence interview" was described by Robert Pynoos, MD. This technique engages the child in drawing and story telling to explore the traumatic experience and to serve as a source of insight into the child's emotional response. The information from the drawings and stories identifies areas in which emotional support and coping skills for the child and family could be provided. The use of drawings and story telling is now widely recognized as a simple but powerful method of communication with children. Play therapy uses games, puppets, clay, and photographs. Play therapy can also be used to break through communication barriers with children traumatized by violence.

Critical incident stress debriefing has been used very successfully for adults, especially out-of-hospital care workers, subsequent to particularly violent or emotional experiences. The techniques of CISD can be applied to children either individually or in classroom settings. Psychological first aid (PFA), as described by Drs Pynoos and Nader, details steps for PFA according to age and grade level in school. An EMS-C targeted-issues grant developed a PFA-like model that combines drawing and story telling with principles of CISD. The focus of this model is early identification of children who have been exposed to violence and the provision of coping skills to the children and their families with follow-up and mental-health referral for children with continued problems. A team approach utilizes an adolescent member for age and cultural sensitivity, paramedics for their CISD background and experience, and mental-health professionals. This PFA model utilizes an activity book titled *Let's Talk about Living in a World of Violence* by James Garbarino. It is available in both English and Spanish. More information on this book can be obtained on the Internet at Web site http://cornell.child.edu.

Psychological first aid is an important mental-health component of EMS-C. Mental health–related objectives are integral to the EMS-C Five Year Plan published by the Health Resources and Services Administration (HRSA) and the National Highway Traffic Safety Administration (NHTSA) and are listed in Table 4. Bibliographies of research publications and intervention programs can be identified through Internet Web sites such as the Domestic Abuse Project (DAP) at http://www.umn.edu/mincava/bibs/bibkids. In addition, resource lists of child-oriented booklets on PTSD and grief are available on the Internet. For help in identifying and accessing information from the Internet see Chapter 9, "Available On-Line Resources."

Table 4.

Mental-Health Objectives From the EMS-C Five Year Plan

•••

- Increase the number of emergency departments that use injury follow-up guidelines to reduce the risk-taking behavior of children, adolescents, and their families
- Increase the number of hospitals that provide or arrange follow-up mental-health services for children and adolescents treated for self-destructive behavior

•••

Summary

A large number of children witness violence each year, placing them at risk for development of PTSD and other mental-health problems. These children need to be identified early through screening and provided with specialized mental-health services. Pediatricians play an important role in the process of identification and referral.

Suggested Reading

Groves BM, Zuckerman B, Marans S, Cohen DJ. Silent victims: children who witness violence. *JAMA.* 1993;269:262–264

Johnson K. *Trauma in the Lives of Children: Crisis and Stress Management Techniques for Teachers, Counselors, and Student Service Professionals.* Claremont, CA: Hunter House; 1989

Knapp JF. The impact of children witnessing violence. *Pediatr Clin North Am.* 1998;45:355–364

Lystad M, ed. *Violence in the Home: Interdisciplinary Perspectives.* New York, NY: Brunner/Mazel; 1986:193–216

Pynoos RS, Eth S. Special intervention programs for child witnesses to violence. In: Pynoos RS, Nader K. Psychological first aid and treatment approach to children exposed to community violence: research implications. *J Traumatic Stress.* 1988;1:445–473

Zuckerman B, Augustyn M, Groves BM, Parker S. Silent victims revisited: the special case of domestic violence. *Pediatrics.* 1995;96:511–513

Resources

Heegaard ME. *When Someone Very Special Dies: Can Children Learn to Cope with Grief.* Minneapolis, MN: Woodland Press; 1988

Garbarino J. *Let's Talk about Living in a World of Violence: An Activity Book for School-Age Children.* Chicago, IL: Erikson Institute; 1993

Part II
....

Office Preparation

....

Although most visits to the primary care physician are scheduled and planned, emergencies in the office do arise. A great deal of information has become available in the past decade regarding the process 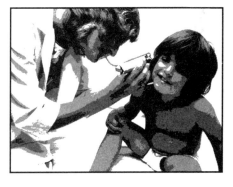 of preparing the office for emergencies. The frequency of emergencies in the office may vary by practice, but the need to be able to act appropriately in a timely manner with proper equipment readily available is universal. In the "pain free" office, for example, sedation and analgesia require special preparation. Extensive on-line resources are available, and this part of the book can become a frequently used reference. It deals with preparing the office for pediatric emergency care.

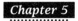

Preparing the Medical Home for Emergencies

Key Points for Office Preparedness

1. Children who require emergency treatment present on an average of weekly to the office.

2. The office is an important component of EMS-C.

3. All office staff should participate in preparation for emergencies.

4. Essential, desirable, and optional equipment lists are available.

Introduction

Do pediatricians encounter and manage emergencies in their offices? Are they adequately prepared? Consider the following scenarios. It is a particularly busy early afternoon in the office. You stopped at the hospital after lunch to make rounds on your patients, and your nurse and receptionist are alone at the office, expecting your return, and the waiting room is already crowded. A 15-month-old boy who is waiting to be seen for a well-child visit suddenly begins to choke, turns blue, and stops breathing. His mother cries out that he had put something in his mouth just prior to the event. The office oxygen tank is empty. Is your office ready and prepared to handle this emergency? A 3-week-old infant has been brought to your office for evaluation of poor feeding and vomiting. At a glance, she is observed to be pale and mottled. Would your receptionist have recognized this emergency and taken appropriate action?

Children who are critically ill or injured will be brought to the pediatric office for emergency care. Children who are a part of your medical home will be seriously injured, have airway obstruction, take life-threatening toxic substances, experience respiratory failure or shock from a variety of causes, or have any number of serious injury events that may threaten life and limb. When these events occur, children are dependent on a system of out-of-hospital emergency care that must address the special needs of children. The medical home must be prepared for emergencies and be an integral part of the EMS-C continuum.

Office emergencies are not a rare event. If an emergency is defined as a patient who requires emergency treatment or subsequent emergency hospitalization, the average pediatrician sees more than two emergencies per week. Surveys of pediatric practice reveal that preparation of the office and staff to respond to the emergency needs of infants and children is not complicated, is not costly, and reduces the stress level of the physician and office staff when critical events occur. Data confirm that most pediatricians are quite skilled in managing critical pediatric emergencies in an emergency department setting, but many are uncomfortable caring for those same problems in an office practice environment. Fortunately, the most life-threatening emergencies rarely present to the office. When an emergency occurs, there is no time for detailed preparation; so the necessary skills, equipment, and plans to address such potentially disastrous situations must be anticipated.

The medical home is an entry point for emergency care and must be a part of the system of emergency care. EMS-C refers not only to ambulance services, but also to all out-of-hospital care, emergency stabilization, trauma services, pediatric emergency specialty care, interfacility transport, inpatient and intensive care, and rehabilitation services. The focal point for these services is the medical home. This chapter focuses on that small but essential component of EMS-C, *the office practice.* Be mindful, however, that preparation of the office cannot be done in isolation. Part of office practice preparation is having knowledge of the capabilities of out-of-hospital systems and access to inpatient and critical specialty services. It also includes training families to be prepared should an emergency occur (see Chapter 3).

The North Carolina EMS-C project prepared a manual called *Office Preparedness for Pediatric Emergencies.* The manual concentrates on recognizing emergencies, preparing a response plan, equipment, physician skills, maintaining readiness, and documentation. It contains model protocols and algorithms, in addition to equipment lists. A single copy of *Office Preparedness for Pediatric Emergencies* can be obtained from the National EMS-C Resource Center free of charge. See the Resources section at the end of this chapter for details.

The Spectrum of Office Emergencies

If the office is to be prepared for pediatric emergencies, the physician must be able to anticipate problems. Preparation should be directed toward management of those emergencies most likely to be encountered. Severe asthma and respiratory distress are the most common emergencies identified by the AAP survey. Seizures, shock (severe dehydration, sepsis, anaphylaxis), and airway obstruction also are common. Cardiac arrest and severe trauma are seen on occasion.

Preparation of an office for emergencies depends on the spectrum of patients receiving care. Preparation for rural practices may differ from that for suburban or urban practices (see Chapter 17). Specialty services that address children with special healthcare needs, such as allergy and cardiac treatment, and children who are technologically assisted may require more extensive skills, equipment, and drugs. The typical primary-care pediatric office practice should be prepared to stabilize children presenting with respiratory distress, respiratory failure, seizures, and shock. The ability to recognize these entities early, provide stabilization, and access safe and efficient transport and definitive care serves as an indicator of office preparedness.

Triage

Triage is the process of sorting patients according to the urgency of their medical needs. Three aspects of triage should be a part of every emergency-ready office practice:

- Predetermined guidelines identifying conditions that will be managed in the office rather than in an emergency department
- Telephone triage guidelines
- Staff triage of patients who arrive at the office for care

Conditions that can be treated in an office setting and those that should be referred directly to an emergency department should be clearly defined and understood by all office staff. These guidelines will vary depending on the special needs of patients seen and the availability of referral resources. Having guidelines in place will facilitate prearrival triage and may avoid unnecessary and risky emergency visits to the office setting.

Write or obtain specific telephone screening guidelines. Every office depends on secretaries, receptionists, and nurses to screen calls during office hours. Many primary-care physicians use nursing staff to screen calls at night. All persons must be adequately instructed to make an appropriate telephone decision regarding a patient's disposition. Office personnel should be instructed to determine if a true emergency exists when a call is received. Clear guidelines should be in place, and the specific actions to be taken by office personnel in case of an emergency should be delineated.

Several excellent references on telephone triage present an organized approach to sorting patients by history obtained during a telephone encounter (see Suggested Reading at the end of this chapter). Because parents and patients are often instructed to contact their primary-care physician first in an emergency, emergency calls are often triaged through the office practice. Personnel answering the telephone must be instructed to never place a patient on "hold" until it is determined that an emergency does not exist. Representatives from the telephone company can provide useful information to office personnel that will help to assess the performance of the existing telephone system. Local telephone companies can provide information that may predict the busiest telephone hours and the frequency of *busy signals* obtained during peak periods. This information can be useful in determining whether additional telephone lines are necessary to assist all families that need help. Emergency telephone numbers and brief protocols that will enable office personnel to give parents prearrival instructions for emergencies such as airway obstruction, uncontrolled bleeding, and seizures are important components of office guidelines. They also improve the consistency of information given during a crisis.

Often the person with the least medical training (the receptionist) is put in the position of making triage decisions in a busy office practice. The receptionist may be required to maintain surveillance on a busy waiting room and determine the need for emergency care. The receptionist should be trained to recognize early signs of shock, respiratory distress and failure, and altered levels of consciousness. The receptionist should be trained to make three quick observations that will identify most potentially serious emergencies. These observations include assessment of the skin, ventilatory system, and appearance (see Table 5). A receptionist trained to observe and assess these situations should be able to identify most infants and children requiring early intervention.

Table 5.
Tips for Preparing for Office Emergencies: Three Quick Receptionist Observations for Identifying Potentially Serious Emergencies

1. **Skin:** Look for pallor, blueness, mottling, and petechiae (spots for identifying signs of shock and sepsis).
2. **Ventilation:** Look at respiratory rate and work of breathing (retractions, nasal flaring, head bobbing) to identify signs of respiratory distress and failure.
3. **Appearance:** Look for altered behavior that does not fit the age of the child.

Staff Preparation

The AAP advocates basic life support (BLS) training for every parent, yet office practice surveys have demonstrated that 75% of office receptionists are not trained in BLS. Data also suggest that pediatric advanced life support (PALS) is not considered a priority for most office physicians and nursing staff. Excellent courses in BLS are available through the American Heart Association (AHA) and the Red Cross (see Chapter 2). Train all office staff in basic cardiopulmonary resuscitation (CPR), including management of the obstructed airway, chest compressions, and ventilatory support.

All office practices and clinics should have personnel on duty who are trained in PALS or CPR (RN or MD). Recent surveys have shown that fewer than 40% of physicians and fewer than 10% of nurses working in office practices have PALS training. CPR courses are readily available in most communities. PALS is available through the AAP and the AHA, and APLS is available through the AAP and American College of Emergency Physicians (ACEP). Both courses are continually updated, have professional surveillance, and train healthcare physicians in skills that will allow them to be comfortable and organized when crises arise (see Chapter 2).

Mock code drills are an excellent method for preparing staff to work together in an organized fashion during a crisis. Chapter 2 contains information on training for mock codes and sample mock-code scenarios. The *Office Preparedness for Pediatric Emergencies* manual also contains a section on using mock codes in the office. Mock codes provide a method for the staff to remain current on how to access equipment, to work together as a team in an emergency, and to practice life-saving protocols in an organized fashion. Routine use of mock codes to sharpen and maintain skills should be a part of every office emergency preparedness program. Receptionists and clerical staff should be a part of this process.

Organizing the Office

Equipment, Supplies, and Drugs

Tables 6 and 7 list equipment, supplies, and drugs recommended for an emergency-prepared office. No one list can possibly serve as an accurate, comprehensive resource that will meet the needs of every office practice. The drugs, equipment, and supplies listed in Tables 6 and 7 are categorized as *essential*, *strongly suggested*, or *optional*. The precise needs of each office setting will vary, and lists serve only as guidelines for preparation. Essential equipment, supplies, and drugs are those most likely to be needed to provide life-saving interventions in the first 10 minutes of an emergency event. No matter what available resources to care for emergencies exist, every office practice should have essential items to provide life support. Strongly suggested and optional equipment, drugs, and supplies may vary among practices.

Most urban and suburban practices can access an EMS system and obtain help within 10 minutes. Nearly 90% of practices are within 5 miles of a community emergency department. A general pediatric practice that can access paramedics skilled in pediatric resuscitation in less than 10 minutes and have its patient at an emergency department within 20 minutes will likely make use of only those *essential* equipment and supply items identified in Tables 6 and 7. Rural practices with potentially less skilled or available systems may need to take greater responsibility for the stabilization of patients who are critically ill prior to transport to definitive care. There are no data that dictate precisely what is necessary for emergency stabilization in each setting; so good judgment must be exercised when choosing proper drugs, equipment, and supplies.

Table 6.

Office Emergency Drugs

Drug	Priority*
Albuterol for inhalation†	E
Epinephrine (1:1000)	E
Activated charcoal	S
Antibiotics	S
Anticonvulsants (Diazepam/Lorazepam)	S
Corticosteroids (parenteral/oral)	S
Dextrose (25%)	S
Diphenhydramine (parenteral, 50 mg/ml)	S
Epinephrine (1:10,000)	S
Atropine sulfate (0.1 mg/ml)	O
Ipecac	O
Naloxone (0.4 mg/ml)	O
Sodium bicarbonate (4.2%)	O
IV Fluids:	
Normal saline or lactated Ringer's (500-ml bags)	O
5% Dextrose, 0.45 NS (500-ml bags)	O

*E, essential; S, strongly suggested; O, optional.
†Metered-dose inhaler with spacer or mask may be substituted.

Table 7.

Office Emergency Equipment and Supplies

Airway	*Priority**
Oxygen and delivery system	E
Bag-valve-mask (450 ml and 1000 ml)	E
Clear oxygen masks, breather and non-rebreather, with reservoirs (infant, child, adult)	E
Suction device, tonsil tip, bulb syringe	E
Peak flow meter	E
Nebulizer (or metered-dose inhaler with spacer/mask)	E
Oral airways (sizes 00–5)	E
Nasal airways (sizes 12–30f)	S
Magill forceps (pediatric, adult)	S
Suction catheters (sizes 5–14f)	S
Nasogastric tubes (sizes 6–14f)	S
Pulse oximeter	S
Laryngoscope handle (pediatric, adult) with extra batteries, bulbs	S
Laryngoscope blades (straight 0–4; curved 2–3)	S
Endotracheal tubes (uncuffed 2.5–5.5; cuffed 6.0–8.0)	S
Stylets (pediatric, adult)	S

Fluid Management	
Butterfly needles (19–25 ga)	S
Catheter-over-needle device (14–24 ga)	S
Arm boards, tape, tourniquet	S
Intraosseous needles (16, 18 ga)	S
Intravenous tubing, microdrip	S

Miscellaneous Equipment and Supplies	
Color-coded tape or preprinted drug doses	E
Cardiac arrest board/backboard	E
Sphygmomanometer (infant, child, adult, thigh cuffs)	E
Splints, sterile dressings	E
Spot glucose test	S
Stiff neck collars (small/large)	S

*E, essential; S, strongly suggested; O, optional.

All office physicians and nursing staff should be skilled in bag-valve-mask ventilation techniques. The skill of endotracheal intubation is not always necessary when there is ready access to definitive pediatric emergency care. Likewise, vascular access and fluid and drug delivery are usually not necessary when advanced resuscitation support is available in less than 10 minutes. Anticonvulsants can be given by the rectal (diazepam) or intramuscular (midazolam) routes if vascular access is not available. Magill forceps for life-saving removal of foreign bodies from the airway must be used with a proper laryngoscope and blade. These instruments are placed in the "strongly suggested" category because they are rarely needed, but they are equally necessary in an urban or rural practice setting. Oxygen saturation obtained by pulse oximetry provides extremely useful information in an office that provides routine nebulizer care for asthmatics. If a pulse oximeter is not available in the office for use in emergencies, the patient should be placed on oxygen with the use of a non-rebreathing oxygen reservoir mask pending transport to definitive care.

Policies and Protocols

Fewer than half of pediatricians have written protocols that guide management of common pediatric emergencies. Although written policies, protocols, and procedures do not ensure an emergency-prepared pediatric office, a manual that includes such information should be a component of every emergency-prepared office practice. This manual serves as a reference to support mock codes, the preparation of emergency equipment and supplies, and the organization of staff in an emergency. An office emergency manual should include:

- Specific algorithms for managing office emergencies to include *at least* stabilization of airway and breathing problems, shock, and seizures
- Lists of emergency equipment and supplies with expiration dates to ensure that outdated drugs and all equipment and supplies are replaced in a timely fashion (one staff member should be responsible for equipment and supplies)
- Instructions on how to access the EMS system and obtain emergency poison information

- Emergency decision-making protocols to be used *when the physician is not in the office*
- Prearranged agreements with an emergency department equipped and staffed to manage pediatric emergencies and with a pediatric intensive care unit to accept patients at the time of an emergency
- Policies for the types of emergencies that may be treated in an office versus those that must go directly to the emergency department
- Precise instructions for managing potential emergencies in regard to office patients who have special healthcare needs or chronic problems that enable the practitioner to anticipate and be prepared for expected emergencies
- Policies for managing children with advanced directives (do not resuscitate)

Facility Preparation

One area of the office should be designated for managing critically ill or injured children. This area should be easily accessible to ambulance and EMS personnel. Equipment and supplies should be readily accessible in this area and organized in such a way that little thought need be given to calculating drug dosages and selecting equipment size at the time of an emergency. Color coding drug doses, equipment, and supplies utilizing a length-based system (Broselow tape) can facilitate the correct choice of emergency equipment and allow the pediatrician to concentrate on more critical management issues. Oxygen delivery devices should be organized and prepared for immediate use. Suction should always be ready with appropriate catheters and suction equipment prepared for emergency use. Physicians and nursing staff should be well skilled in providing bag-valve-mask ventilation and in using the appropriate technique to ensure emergency ventilation of the infant or child with respiratory failure.

Summary

Time spent in organizing the resuscitation area and ensuring that staff know how to access management protocols and the appropriate equipment, supplies, and drugs will reduce stress and improve outcome when emergencies arise. Advance preparation by developing emergency protocols, training staff, and organizing emergency supplies can reduce stress and support the medical home as a part of the EMS-C continuum.

Suggested Reading

Altieri M, Bellet J, Scott H. Preparedness for pediatric emergencies encountered in the practitioner's office. *Pediatrics.* 1990;85:710–714

American Academy of Pediatrics Department of Research. Periodic survey of fellows #27: emergency readiness in pediatric offices. Elk Grove Village, IL: American Academy of Pediatrics; June 1995

Flores G, Weinstock DJ. The preparedness of pediatricians for emergencies in the office: what is broken, should we care, and how can we fix it? *Arch Pediatr Adolesc Med.* 1996;150:249–256

Fuchs S, Jaffe DM, Christoffel KK. Pediatric emergencies in office practices: prevalence and office preparedness. *Pediatrics.* 1989;83:931–939

Hodge D 3rd. Pediatric emergency office equipment. *Pediatr Emerg Care.* 1988;4:212–214

Katz, HP. *Telephone Medicine: Triage and Training, A Handbook for Primary Health Care Professionals.* 2nd ed. Thorofare, NJ: Slack, Incorporated; 1990

Katz, HP. Telephone medicine. In: Dershewitz RA, ed. *Ambulatory Pediatric Care.* 2nd ed. Philadelphia, PA: J. B. Lippincott Company; 1993:6–9

Lubitz DS, Seidel JS, Chameides L, Luten RC, Zaritsky AL, Campbell FW. A rapid method for estimating weight and resuscitation drug dosages from length in the pediatric age group. *Ann Emerg Med.* 1988;17:576–581

Schmitt B. *Pediatric Telephone Advice: Guidelines for the Health Care Physician on Telephone Triage and Office Management of Common Childhood Symptoms.* Boston, MA: Little, Brown; 1980

Schweich PJ, DeAngelis C, Duggan AK. Preparedness of practicing pediatricians to manage emergencies. *Pediatrics.* 1991;88:223–229

Seidel J. Preparing for pediatric emergencies. *Pediatr Rev.* 1995;16:466–472

Resources

Selected AAP resources include:

Drugs for Pediatric Emergencies

First Aid Chart

Descriptions and ordering information are available at the AAP Web site at http://www.aap.org

Other related resources are in the AAP Publications Resource List at the end of this manual

Office Preparedness for Pediatric Emergencies: Physician Manual can be obtained by accessing the National EMS-C Resource Center home page at http://www.ems-c.org and clicking on EMS-C Publications and Products. Or you may request this publication by using the four-digit code 0614 and writing, calling, or e-mailing:

EMS-C Clearinghouse
2070 Chain Bridge Road
Suite 450
Vienna, VA 22182-2536
Telephone: (703) 902-1203
Fax: (703) 821-2098
E-mail: emsc@circsol.com

Analgesia and Sedation in the Office

Introduction

Children deserve effective management of pain and anxiety during procedures. Advantages of providing analgesia and sedation include relief from pain and reduction of distress during present and future interactions with healthcare providers, reduction of parental and physician distress, and improved performance of procedures. Office management of painful procedures incorporates preprocedure preparation of the child and parents, comforting and distraction during the procedure, and administration of local or systemic analgesics and, occasionally, light sedation.

Preprocedure Preparation

Preparation for procedures includes decreasing anxiety for parents and children. Younger children require simple language and visual explanations (eg, hands-on demonstrations with dolls), whereas older children understand more detailed information. Understanding and addressing patients' perceptions and feelings about procedures and providing information about what will be done and what it may feel like are essential. Brief explanations of what may (or may not) hurt, how much it may hurt, and when the hurting will stop can help patients prepare. For example, age-appropriate empathetic explanations of imminent needle sticks have been shown to reduce crying compared with impersonal instructions. Discussion of procedural pain too far in advance or dwelling extensively on impending pain, however, may heighten anxiety and lower patients' tolerance for discomfort. After a brief description of the procedure, assure patients that they will be warned before something may hurt and empower them to control their pain by using relaxation, distraction, or self-hypnosis, and so forth. Distractions such as playful interactions during explanations, maintaining patient eye contact, sitting during explanations, and allowing time for questions help establish trust and reduce anxiety. Addressing parental questions and concerns also helps parents aid their children during the process. Finally, acceptable behavior should be established with the child before the procedure begins.

Parental Presence

Parental presence during painful procedures is desired by virtually all children and most parents, yet it has been shown to be inconsistent in reducing children's distress. It is important to assess the nature of the parents' relation with their children, their own level of distress about the medical procedure, and their ability to enhance or their potential to interfere with their children's abilities to cope. A positive correlation has been found between parental anxiety and children's distress during bone marrow aspiration. Distress can be significantly reduced by suggesting techniques such as touching, story telling, or imagery. Informed parents rarely interfere with the performance of the procedure. Preparation should be made for the possibility of parental distress or syncope during the procedure.

Comforting and Distraction

Nonpharmacologic techniques such as relaxation, distraction, and imagery reduce procedural pain and distress in many children. **Relaxation** for infants or young children may consist simply of rocking, swaddling, or holding the children in comfortable, well-supported positions. Allowing sucking or providing something to grasp also may reduce distress. With older children, deep breaths during a procedure with slow inhalation and exhalation to "blow away the pain" can be effective. Blowing soap bubbles can be distracting and evolve into a relaxation technique with slow rhythmic breathing. Ideally, these techniques are taught prior to the procedure and used to reduce distress both before and during the procedure. Whether the demonstrated efficacy of these techniques results from distraction from the painful stimulus, stimulation of larger afferent tracks that interfere with pain transmission, or effects of vestibular stimulation is unknown.

Distraction focuses patients' attention on a diversion to put their pain and distress at the periphery of their awareness. Distraction can be accomplished without special equipment by engaging children of all ages in a variety of tasks, such as focusing attention on objects in the room, singing, counting, and story telling. Inexpensive tape recorders and children's tapes are popular. A more expensive option is to have one room equipped with a television, videocassette recorder, and CD player. Developmental consideration and individual interests are important in developing effective distraction techniques. Allowing children and parents to identify what is particularly interesting to them improves distraction and grants them some control in the procedure.

Imagery employs the development of pleasant scenes, actions, hobbies, favorite television programs, movies, and so forth, into fantasies. It may be as simple as picturing themselves elsewhere or doing something fun. Story telling can be developed into imagery by incorporating the sensory experience of the procedure. Developmental consideration and individual interests are essential in developing effective imagery techniques.

Children between 2 and 7 years of age will likely have difficulty understanding the reasons for medical procedures. Attempts to reason with very young children are usually not helpful. These children may benefit more from play therapy before the procedure and simple distraction techniques and reinforcement of positive behaviors during the procedure. Younger children and those with developmental delay may do better with behavioral techniques that require less cognitive effort such as conversation, visual distractions, and counting. Pictures can be placed on the ceiling to effectively divert the child's attention. Structured strategies for toddlers include pop-up books and toys, blowing bubbles, looking through a kaleidoscope, and watching videos. Pop-up books and toys provide multiple novel stimuli that help capture and recapture children's attention whenever they start to focus on the painful procedure. Age-appropriate activities for preschool children include videos, searching for objects in pictures, blowing away pain, and superhero imagery or other story telling.

Children 8 years and older likely can understand reasons for procedures and respond to distraction. Listening to music or a story through a headset or watching a video can be highly effective. Singing aloud a familiar song and keeping time to the music is another simple distraction. Counting and imagery are also helpful in this age group. Adolescents may regress when they become acutely anxious and may require help in using effective coping mechanisms. Discussion of the procedures with plans for coping and practice of coping techniques can be quite useful.

Equipment and Supply Preparation

All equipment needed should be readied so that the procedure can be accomplished efficiently. Such equipment includes appropriately sized airways, a bag-valve-mask ventilator and oxygen, suctioning, and appropriate pharmacologic reversal agents. Preparing equipment out of view may lessen children's anxiety. Many children may understand a detailed examination and explanation of the equipment, but this should not delay beginning the procedure.

Pharmacologic Interventions

The relief of pain for procedures can be accomplished effectively and safely in a primary-care office by using local anesthesia, oral analgesia, and distraction techniques. The use of oral sedatives to induce light or conscious sedation should be judicious and "carry a margin of safety wide enough to render unintended loss of consciousness highly unlikely" (AAP sedation guidelines; see the Resources section at the end of this chapter). Because few medications have such a margin of safety and individual patient response to sedatives can vary unpredictably and because unintended deep sedation is difficult to manage, procedures performed in the office are generally accomplished without pharmacologic sedation.

Local Anesthetics

EMLA, a eutectic mixture of local anesthetics (lidocaine and prilocaine) in a cream formulation applied under occlusion for 60 minutes, has been shown to significantly decrease the pain of intravenous catheter placement, accessing subcutaneous vascular ports, lumbar puncture, curettage of molluscum contagiosum, circumcision, and, recently, suturing of extremity wounds and intramuscular immunizations. EMLA cream should not be used on mucous membranes, for patients with a tendency toward methemoglobinemia, or for patients under the age of 12 months who are being treated with methemoglobin-inducing drugs (eg, sulfonamides, acetaminophen, and phenytoin).

TAC and LET solutions and gels containing tetracaine, adrenaline, and cocaine (TAC) or lidocaine, epinephrine, and tetracaine (LET) reduce the pain of suturing when they are applied to the wound for 20 to 30 minutes. These preparations work better on short lacerations of the head and face than on extremity or truncal wounds. Neither of these preparations is commercially available, however, and must be specially prepared by a pharmacist. The TAC preparation also requires strict control because of its cocaine content. Use of these preparations is contraindicated on mucous membranes and large abrasions because of increased absorption with systemic toxicity and on digits and other areas with end arteriolar blood supply (eg, nose, fingers, or penis).

Lidocaine provides local anesthesia with minimal discomfort when buffered with sodium bicarbonate to near-physiologic pH and slowly injected subcutaneously with a 27- or 30-gauge needle. Buffered lidocaine can be prepared by mixing 1 ml of 8.4% sodium bicarbonate (1 mEq/ml) with each 9–10 ml of 1% lidocaine. Shielding the needle from sight and using distraction during injection of buffered lidocaine can result in nearly painless anesthesia for suturing (especially if topical anesthetics are applied first); intravenous catheter placement, lumbar puncture, soft-tissue foreign-body removal, and other procedures are facilitated by local anesthesia. Remember that an overdose of lidocaine may precipitate seizures. A guideline for the maximum dose is 5 mg/kg without epinephrine and 7 mg/kg with epinephrine.

Iontophoresis of 2% lidocaine with epinephrine for 10 to 20 minutes provides effective local anesthesia for venous catheter placement, lumbar puncture, accessing subcutaneous vascular ports, and other procedures facilitated by superficial local anesthesia. Tingling or burning sensations at the electrodes may be uncomfortable for some patients. Commercial products that facilitate iontophoresis (eg, Numby Stuff) have recently become available.

Oral Analgesics

Oral analgesics can significantly reduce postprocedural or injury pain. They can be particularly effective in reducing the pain of fractures and muscular or ligamentous strain or sprains when used along with immobilization of the injured body part.

Acetaminophen acts on nonpiod receptors in the central nervous system (CNS) to inhibit prostaglandin synthesis and undergoes hepatic metabolism and renal excretion. It has no anti-inflammatory effects. Therapeutic doses are rarely associated with side effects, but overdose can cause hepatic toxicity. At an oral dose of 15 mg/kg/dose every 4 hours, it has an onset of effect in 20 to 40 minutes, with a peak effect in 2 hours. Dosing usually should not exceed 90 mg/kg/day or 4–6 g/day.

Aspirin reduces pain through inhibition of prostaglandin production and has anti-inflammatory effects. Aspirin inhibits platelet function, which can lead to excessive bleeding. Other side effects include gastrointestinal irritation, nausea, vomiting, and bronchospasm in asthmatics. Reye syndrome has been associated with the use of aspirin for varicella and flu-like illness. Overdose may cause reversible liver toxicity and CNS problems such as tinnitus and dizziness. The oral or rectal dose of aspirin is 10–15 mg/kg administered every 4 hours with a maximum of 65 mg/kg/day. Buffered aspirin may be better tolerated and absorbed faster, but there is no evidence that it acts more rapidly or lasts longer. Enteric-coated aspirin is better tolerated but has variable absorption.

Ibuprofen, tolmetin, ketorolac, and naproxen are nonsteroidal anti-inflammatory drugs (NSAIDs) that have a longer half-life and are thought to be more potent than aspirin. These drugs are particularly of value in treating pain of musculoskeletal origin and dysmenorrhea. They act on the peripheral nervous system to block formation of prostaglandins. Adverse effects associated with NSAIDs include platelet dysfunction, hepatic toxicity, water retention, hyperkalemia, hypertension, renal dysfunction, and gastrointestinal toxicity. In contrast with aspirin, the effect on platelets is reversible. NSAIDs have cross-reactivity with aspirin and should not be used for patients who have aspirin sensitivity. Because they may cause gastrointestinal symptoms such as dyspepsia, bleeding, and ulceration, NSAIDs should be taken with meals. Ketorolac is indicated for short-term (up to 5 days) management of moderately severe pain. However, efficacy and safety in children younger than 16 years old have not been established. Ketorolac may also be given intramuscularly to selected patients. In addition, safety and efficacy for naproxen have not been established in children younger than 2 years old.

Narcotic Analgesics

Oral narcotics are useful for severe or moderately severe pain. Opioid analgesics include the naturally occurring compounds morphine and codeine as well as the synthetic agonists with morphine-like activity. All narcotics exert their effects through reversible binding with both CNS and peripheral endorphin and enkephalin receptors. Binding and stimulation of these receptors decreases pain sensation and general awareness. Although all narcotics depress respiratory drive to some degree, there are minimal ventilatory depressive effects with therapeutic doses of orally administered narcotics. More common adverse reactions associated with orally administered narcotics include nausea, vomiting, smooth muscle spasm, constipation, and urinary retention.

Codeine is given orally because it maintains two-thirds of its effectiveness in oral form. Approximately 10% of codeine is metabolized into morphine and is responsible for the analgesic effects. Approximately 10% of the population cannot metabolize codeine into morphine and, in these patients, codeine will have no analgesic effects. Codeine can cause respiratory depression, but this effect is rare. It has no renal or hepatic toxicity and does not alter platelet function, but it often causes nausea and other adverse gastrointestinal effects.

Oxycodone is a semisynthetic analogue of codeine. It may cause less nausea and vomiting and is ten times as potent as codeine and about equal to morphine in potency. Like codeine, it retains more than half of its efficacy when given orally. It is often combined with aspirin (Percodan) or acetaminophen (Percocet, Tylox) to potentiate the analgesic effects. The analgesic takes effect as early as 20 minutes after dosing and reaches a maximum at 60–120 minutes. The plasma half-life is from 2.5 to 4 hours.

Codeine and oxycodone are available in liquid, tablet, and capsule forms. Typically, codeine is prescribed in a dose of 0.5–1.0 mg/kg every 4 hours and oxycodone in a dose of 0.05–0.1 mg/kg every 6 hours. Codeine and acetaminophen are commonly prescribed as "numbered" tablets with tablet number 1 containing 7.5 mg of codeine, number 2 containing 15 mg, number 3 containing 30 mg, and number 4 containing 60 mg. Acetaminophen and codeine elixirs contain 120 mg of acetaminophen and 12 mg of codeine, respectively, per teaspoon. Oxycodone liquid is available in a 1-mg/ml concentration.

Transmucosyl fentanyl, the Oralet, is available in 100-, 200-, 300-, and 400-mcg sizes. The dose is 10–15 mcg/kg. It should not be used in children who weigh less than 15 kg. It should be administered only in a monitored setting and is not for home use. Oxygen desaturation can occur with the use of this agent and postsedation nausea and vomiting has been reported.

Benzodiazepines

Midazolam is a water-soluble benzodiazepine with sedative, anxiolytic, and amnestic properties but provides no analgesia. When the intravenous solution is administered orally in a dose of 0.2–0.5 mg/kg, mild anxiolysis and sedation are achieved after 15 to 30 minutes, with recovery typically within an hour after administration. Because of its bitter taste, the solution is usually mixed with flavoring such as cherry, grape, or chocolate syrup, orange juice, or acetaminophen suspension. Occasionally, agitated dysphoria or disinhibition results. Intranasal administration of the intravenous solution, 0.2–0.4 mg/kg, results in more rapid onset of effects but causes a burning sensation in some patients. Young children and infants may prefer rectal administration of the solution, 0.5 mg/kg. Significant respiratory depression rarely occurs when midazolam is administered without concurrent use of opioids or other sedatives, but patients should be continuously monitored for this adverse effect.

Nitrous Oxide

Dentists have used nitrous oxide in the out-patient management of pain for years with few reports of adverse cardiopulmonary effects. It provides amnesia, anxiolysis, and from mild to moderate analgesia when administered at a concentration of 50% mixed with 50% oxygen. Common side effects at this dose include vomiting, dizziness, and headache. Although the equipment may be costly initially, it is easy to use. Oxygen saturation and heart rate should be continuously monitored when delivering nitrous oxide. Nitrous oxide should not exceed 50% in the office setting and should be administered only by physicians who are familiar with the agent and with cardiopulmonary resuscitation and who have appropriate resuscitation equipment immediately available. Nitrous oxide should not be combined with any other sedating agent, because it may result in deep sedation or general anesthesia. Because of the risk of abuse, it should be stored in a controlled area. It should be used with caution in patients with otitis media and is contraindicated in patients with suspected bowel obstruction. The use of nitrous oxide should generally be reserved for the emergency department.

Definition of Sedation

If sedative medications are used, carefully follow the AAP Guidelines for Monitoring of Sedated Patients. Conscious sedation (CS) as defined in these guidelines is a medically controlled state of depressed consciousness that allows protective reflexes to be maintained, retains the patient's ability to maintain a patent airway independently and continuously, and permits appropriate response by the patient to physical stimulation and verbal command (eg, "open your eyes"). Conscious sedation is now used synonymously with the expression "sedation and analgesia." Conscious sedation does not mean reflex response to pain but rather a purposeful response to a painful stimulus, such as patient saying "ouch" when something hurts. Deep sedation (DS) is defined as the level of depressed consciousness or unconsciousness from which the patient is not easily aroused and does not respond purposefully to physical stimulation or verbal command. DS may be accompanied by a partial or complete loss of protective reflexes and the inability to maintain a patent airway independently. CS and DS lie along a continuum anchored at one end by full alertness and reflexes and at the other by general anesthesia. It is often unclear when a patient progresses from CS to DS with its concomitant increased risks for aspiration and respiratory depression.

The AAP Guidelines recommend, for a patient undergoing CS, that the practitioner responsible for the treatment of the patient be trained in sedation techniques, be capable of managing complications of the sedation, and be prepared for unintended progression into DS or obtundation. Obtain training in advanced pediatric life support. An additional person is required to help monitor the patient's physiologic status and to assist in any supportive measures. Continually measure the patient's oxygen saturation, heart rate and respiratory rate, and intermittently record blood pressure. A functioning suction apparatus and equipment to deliver greater than 90% oxygen and assisted ventilation and ventilation (bag-mask apparatus) along with appropriately sized airways should be at the bedside.

Very painful procedures (eg, fracture reduction or burn debridement) often require periods of DS during which the patient is at risk for respiratory depression and aspiration. DS requires that a physician experienced in advanced pediatric life support be at the patient's bedside exclusively to administer the sedative, analgesic, or resuscitative medications and to monitor and support the patient's cardiorespiratory functions during the procedure and postprocedure periods. This person should not be responsible for helping to accomplish the painful procedure. Full cardiopulmonary monitoring is employed and resuscitation equipment needs to be immediately available. DS should be performed only in an emergency department, operating suite, or other area fully equipped and staffed for patient monitoring and resuscitation as outlined in the AAP Guidelines.

Presedation Evaluation, Monitoring, and Discharge

Presedation evaluation before beginning the sedation includes a careful patient history and physical evaluation, with particular attention to the cardiorespiratory status and airway (to determine the ability to rescue breathe for the patient if necessary). Focus your examination on any problems that might lead to difficulties with airway management or compromise the airway once the child is sedated (eg, large tonsils, etc.). Patients who have taken clear liquids from 2 to 3 hours prior to the procedure or solids, breast milk, or formula from 4 to 6 hours prior to it may have increased risk of vomiting and aspiration.

Monitoring is necessary until the patient returns to the presedation level of responsiveness. The support person should continue to closely observe the patient during the recovery period.

A procedure note should include sufficiency of the patient's vital functions (heart rate, respiratory rate, and oxygen saturation) and level of consciousness, time and dose of medications, and description of any complications and interventions.

The patient may be discharged when the vital signs are stable and he or she is alert, able to talk, sit unaided, drink without difficulty, and walk with minimal assistance. For the very young or the handicapped patient for whom this assessment is impossible, the presedation level of responsiveness should be achieved. At discharge, a parental information sheet should be given that reviews potential medication side effects and limitation of unsupervised patient activity, as well as including a telephone number for the parents to call with questions concerning the sedation.

Summary

Effective management of pain and anxiety during procedures can result in relieved and happier patients, parents, and healthcare physicians and improved performance of the procedures. Office management incorporates preprocedure preparation of the children and parents, comforting and distraction during the procedure, local or systemic analgesics, and, occasionally, light sedation.

Suggested Reading

Conway EE, ed. Procedures in the office setting. *Pediatr Ann.* 1996;25 (theme issue):659–704

Ernst AA, Marvez E, Nick TG, Chin E, Wood E, Gonzaba WT. Lidocaine adrenaline tetracaine gel versus tetracaine adrenaline cocaine gel for topical anesthesia in linear scalp and facial lacerations in children aged 5 to 17 years. *Pediatrics.* 1995;95:255–258

Fatovich DM, Jacobs IG. A randomized, controlled trial of oral midazo-lam and buffered lidocaine for suturing lacerations in children (the SLIC Trial). *Ann Emerg Med.* 1995;25:209–214

Gajraj NM, Pennant JH, Watcha MF. Eutectic mixture of local anesthet-ics (EMLA) cream. *Anesth Analg.* 1994;78:574–583

Greenbaum SS, Bernstein EF. Comparison of iontophoresis of lidocaine with a eutectic mixture of lidocaine and prilocaine (EMLA) for topically administered local anesthesia. *J Dermatol Surg Oncol.* 1994;20:579–583

Klein EJ, Shugerman RP, Leigh-Taylor K, Schneider C, Portscheller D, Koepsell T. Buffered lidocaine: analgesia for intravenous line placement in children. *Pediatrics.* 1995;95:709–712

McKay W, Morris R, Mushlin P. Sodium bicarbonate attenuates pain on skin infiltration with lidocaine, with or without epinephrine. *Anesth Analg.* 1987;66:572–574

Rothman KF. Minimizing the pain of office procedures in children. *Curr Opin Pediatr.* 1995;7:415–422

Taddio A, Nulman I, Goldbach M, Ipp M, Koren G. Use of lidocaine-prilocaine cream for vaccination pain in infants. *J Pediatr.* 1994;124:643–648

Resources

American Academy of Pediatrics Committee on Drugs. Guidelines for monitoring and management of pediatric patients during and after sedation for diagnostic and therapeutic procedures. *Pediatrics.* 1992;89:1110–1115

Emergency Services and Managed Care

Key Points in EMS-C and Managed Care

1. Emergency-care provisions should be included in managed-care contracts.

2. The financing of healthcare for children is largely by the government.

3. Children are often cared for by safety-net physicians and hospitals.

4. Pediatricians must advocate insurance plans to provide the most appropriate emergency care for their patients.

Introduction

A healthy 12-year-old presents with acute appendicitis at a hospital 5 miles away. As the admitting physician on call for your hospital, you are called by the medical director of a health management organization (HMO) to arrange for emergency transport to your facility. As you begin to ask a few pertinent clinical questions, the HMO medical director seems annoyed by your questions and reminds you that the HMO is keeping information on every physician in its network. Your report card and your bonus pool could be negatively affected by the appearance of denying or delaying transfer. You arrange transport, and the child subsequently undergoes an operation and is sent home 2 days later. The HMO pays for only a 23-hour observation stay, denies the transport charges, and files a quality-review complaint on you.

This scenario raises several questions about the relation and interaction between physicians and HMOs with regard to EMS-C. Among them are:

1. Why do managed care organizations and EMS-C often appear to be in conflict?
2. How is the financing of insurance for most adults different from that for children?
3. What are some of the issues confronting safety-net physicians?

This chapter attempts to answer these complex questions for the private practitioner. You must become familiar with the definitions of key terms in Table 8. Additional resources are available

Table 8.		

Insurance Financing

Percentage With Each Source of Insurance

Source of Insurance	Adults	Children
Commercial	70%	20%
Government	24%	70% Year 1
		50 % Year 5
Self-pay	6%	10%

through the AAP and the National EMS-C Resource Center (see the Resources section at the end of this chapter).

Differences in Motivation

Physicians who focus on the emergency services of children often spend their time working on issues that are rarely the focus of managed-care organizations. Pediatric physicians are concerned with issues of child advocacy, emergency care for children with special needs, injury prevention, youth violence intervention, and family-centered care. Many pediatric care-givers belong to organizations that are structured as tax-exempt not-for-profit organizations, and, for many of them, achieving break-even status is a challenge.

In contrast, many managed-care organizations (MCOs) are for-profit businesses that must return a profit, in the form of a quarterly dividend check, to the shareholders. Pressure to meet the demands for profit sharing puts pressure on the MCOs to decrease cost, maximize profit, and thereby increase the share-holder wealth. A lower medical loss ratio (MLR) implies that the company can provide care at a lower cost and potentially have more dollars available for the stockholders.

When two large MCOs merged a few years ago, they became responsible for more than 23 million Americans, or 1 in 12 com-mercial lives. They announced to their shareholders that they expected to produce a $300 million profit in the first 18 months, on a total of more than $16 billion of business. The fierce com-petition to achieve such profit margins forces MCOs to decrease their MLRs, and, as a result, many patient services may be sacrificed in the attempt to drive down the cost of care.

Payment by Different Kinds of Insurance

The government is the single largest payer for the health care costs for America's children. In many areas of the United States, more than 60% of the births are covered by Medicaid, and, by year 5 of life, 50% of children are still on some form of government-funded health insurance. Only 20% of children have some form of commercial insurance. Ten percent of children have no insurance and are considered to be in the "self-pay" or "no pay" category. With the advent of the State Child Health Insurance Program (SCHIP;Title XXI), the hope is that some of the children without health insurance will be afforded a Medicaid "clone" or "look-alike" type of insurance.

Because much of the adult work force receives healthcare insurance as part of their work-related benefits, nearly 70% of all adults have some form of commercial insurance (Table 9). Therefore, when MCOs draft policies for their commercial patients, they often do so with the adult patient's needs uppermost. Specialists for coronary artery disease, hip fractures, and Alzheimer disease are more likely to be included on the panel of physicians than are the pediatric subspecialists needed for coarctation of the aorta, congenital hip dysplasias, and attention-deficit disorder.

Table 9.

1996 Medicaid Expenditures by Population

Segment	Number of Patients in the Segment (in Millions)	Percentage of Total Patients	Cost per Segment (in Billions of Dollars)	Percentage of Total Funding
Hospitals			$16.26	12
Elderly	3.65	11	$37.9	28
Blind or disabled	5.36	16	$43.3	32
Adults	7.37	22	$16.2	12
Children	**17.0**	**51**	**$21.6**	**16**

Although many children have good health, and only minor injuries or illnesses from time to time in childhood, 20% of children utilize nearly 80% of the healthcare resources allocated to this age group. This is particularly true of the special-needs populations: the blind, the disabled, the technology dependent, and those with congenital problems. It is this special population, with high resource-utilization needs, that is most at risk of falling through the cracks of typical commercial managed care and even Medicaid managed care. For more information on children with special healthcare needs, see Chapter 15. Because the roots of these conditions are often linked to problems such as poverty, teen pregnancy, and substance abuse, the ability to prevent many of these conditions is limited at best.

Furthermore, 15% of noninstitutionalized Americans, or nearly 37.7 million people, are disabled. Four million of these people are under the age of 18, and more than 690 000 of them have more than one disability. Utilization data reveal that people with disabilities visit a healthcare physician about 10 times a year. In contrast, other than in the first year of life, healthy children rarely have to go to a physician more than once or twice a year, and rarely are they hospitalized.

Another factor that increases the medical vulnerability of children is poverty. One in three children in cities and one in four children in rural areas lives with a family whose income is below the federal poverty line. Forty-five percent of African-American children live in families at or below the federal poverty line. This population is more at risk than those whose incomes are above the poverty line for poor health outcomes and is more dependent on the presence and functioning of their local safety-net physicians to meet its healthcare needs.

Medicaid, a Title XIX entitlement program, provides healthcare benefits for children under 1 year of age in families at less than 185% of the federal poverty line, for children from 1 to 5 years of age in families at less than 133% of the federal poverty line, and for children from 6 to 18 years of age in families at 100% of the federal poverty line. For example, 200% of the federal poverty line in 1997 was $32 100 for a family of four. This entitlement program, with dedicated federal funds, which require obligatory state matching funds, provides more than

$21 billion of care to more than 17 million children. However, this program, as well intentioned as it is, still only spends 16% of its annual budget on children, compared with the remaining 82% spent on the elderly, blind, disabled, and disproportionate-share hospitals (Table 10).

Table 10.

Key Terms in Managed Care

....

1. **Medical loss ratio (MLR).** The ratio of *expenditure* on actual medical care to the *revenue* generated by the insurance premium. An MLR of 82% implies that 82 cents of every premium dollar goes toward the actual care of the patient. The remaining 18 cents goes toward administrative costs, advertising costs, and the profit returned to the owner or investors.
2. **Safety-net physician.** Hospitals and physicians who provide care for children without insurance or children whose insurance is not accepted by certain physicians (Medicaid) or children who have such complex problems that typical community hospitals cannot manage their care are called safety-net physicians.
3. **Title XIX (Medicaid).** A federally funded, requiring state matching funds, entitlement program that provides healthcare benefits for low-income children and some of the elderly and disabled.
4 **Title XXI (the State Child Health Insurance Program (SCHIP).** The 1997 initiative that provides a federal matching program for 5 years (for states that elect to participate) of healthcare benefits for children who fall through the crack between commercial insurance and the federal poverty line requirements for Medicaid.
5. **Capitation.** A prepayment mechanism, based on a per-member-per-month calculation, that covers all the patient's needs, in sickness and in health. Profit is generated by keeping the patient well and out of the hospital, generally through the strict use of primary-care physicians as gatekeepers.

....

Hospitalization in Different Hospitals

Many of the physicians and hospitals that serve the acute and critical needs of children fall into the category of safety-net physicians. Community health centers, public health departments, academic medical centers, county hospitals, and children's hospitals—all are part of the safety net of the most medically vulnerable children in our society.

Because of the higher operating costs associated with some of these facilities, particularly children's hospitals and academic medical centers, many of these traditional safety-net physicians are doomed to extinction in this era of managed competition. If these facilities and their expertise are lost in the managed-care wars, the traditional services provided to the high-risk neonate, the child needing cardiac surgery, the patient awaiting solid organ or bone marrow transplant, the technology-driven ECMO (extracorporeal membrane oxygenation) centers, and the multiply handicapped child may be at risk. Furthermore, as graduate medical education funding is put at greater risk, the ability of academic centers to provide this complex, multispecialty care for the special-needs child is even more endangered.

In an earlier era, when increasing EMS-C might have implied more admissions to a hospital, the hospital administrators might have more readily justified the funding for these services. However, in an era marked by advancing capitation payments, where profits arise from keeping patients out of the hospital and restricting tests, the willingness to provide the high-cost services needed to keep EMS-C care afloat is financially challenged.

If safety-net hospitals and their physicians become jeopardized in the national movements to consolidate hospitals, close units, and decrease length of stay, then emergency departments may become the primary source of care for the underinsured population. Because regulations such as the Emergency Medical Treatment and Active Labor Act (EMTALA/COBRA) protect patients from being turned out of an emergency department without at least a medical-screening examination, emergency departments become by default sometimes the only source of care for this population.

Added to this potential influx of underinsured patients in the emergency department is a mass migration of commercial patients away from emergency departments. Managed-care companies aggressively use nurse telephone triage systems, as well as penalties against primary care physicians, to keep patients out of the emergency department. Although this attempt may be well intentioned, it does drive revenue away from emergency departments, and less money is available to help cover the unmet cost of the medically vulnerable.

When states shift from traditional Medicaid to mandatory Medicaid Managed Care, patients elect or are assigned a primary-care physician. Many of these patients may never have had a strong relation with a primary-care physician ("gatekeeper") prior to their entry into this program. Perhaps they grew up in a community where the emergency department was their primary source of care. This population, when triaged away from emergency departments, may be unfamiliar with or have no access to a nurse telephone triage system. Parents may not be able to miss work to take their children to a primary-care office or health department for a sick-child visit. With this population, managing patients away from the emergency department does not automatically ensure that they are being managed toward a medical home.

Different Systems of Care

Large systems of healthcare are forming throughout the United States after a frenzy of mergers and acquisitions. One hospital chain has more than 350 hospitals and can leverage its size into handsome volume purchasing, driving its costs lower than those of the specialty children's hospital or the stand-alone safety-net physician in the same community. Some of these systems, acting with autocratic efficiency, can narrow the types, brands, and sizes of everything from drinking cups to subclavian catheters nationwide in less than 30 days.

Similarly, physicians' groups are merging or being acquired by for-profit firms. The pressure to decrease the overhead, maximize volume purchasing, increase the number of patients seen per hour, and position for managed-care contracting makes it difficult for the smaller pediatric subspecialties to survive in the marketplace.

Other Considerations in Dealing With Managed Care

- There may be a conflict between federal and state law and the dictates of MCOs. Make MCOs aware of this potential liability to prevent such conflicts.
- Parents can be advocates for their children and primary-care physicians by negotiating with their human resources departments at work and directly with MCOs to ensure access to high-quality emergency care.
- Make sure that your managed-care contract includes access and reimbursement for emergency care.
- Consider all of the implications of the "gate keeping" policies of MCOs and make sure that they are not in conflict with federal or state law or with medical ethics.

Summary

Several points regarding EMS-C and the financing of healthcare should be kept in mind.

1. A conflict often exists between physicians of high-quality EMS-C care and MCOs.
2. The financing of healthcare for children is largely from the government, whereas many adults enjoy the benefits of commercial insurance. Similarly, because few children are covered by commercial insurance, benefit plans often overlook the needs of children in general and those of special-needs children in particular.
3. Safety-net physicians and hospitals often care for children. Many of these institutions are financially threatened by market-driven healthcare reform. Should these facilities close or have to limit services, children may not have access to the same standard of care that they previously enjoyed.
4. Many adult systems are merging and enjoying the benefit of for-profit insurance coverage and the power of group purchasing. Single children's systems and other safety-net physicians are severely disadvantaged by their higher cost structure, the cost of graduate medical education, and the resources used by the child needing multispecialty care.
5. Pediatricians may have to negotiate on behalf of their patients with insurance plans or MCOs in regard to the most appropriate place for their patients to receive emergency care.

All that being said, we are not to lose heart. Other industries have faced similar market challenges. Those that would critically look at themselves and reinvent themselves stood the best chance of surviving the market wars. However, those resistant to change lost out to the winds of change. For example, Swiss watches gave way to Japanese plastic accessory watches. Ford, with a virtual monopoly with the black Model T, created an opportunity for other car makers, because of its slowness in adapting to the market's demand for other colors.

The world of EMS-C is not beyond the reach of market forces. Standing still or resisting change, in this era of market-driven managed competition, ensures consequences. Leaders in EMS-C must plan aggressively, and advocate loudly, for children, whose voices are too quiet to be heard, lest the hard-fought gains in the EMS-C of yesterday be swept away by the market forces of today.

Suggested Reading

American Academy of Pediatrics Committee on Child Health Financing. Guiding principles for managed care arrangements for the health care of infants, children, adolescents, and young adults. *Pediatrics*. 1995;95:613–615

American Academy of Pediatrics Committee on Child Health Financing. Implementation principles and strategies for Title XXI State Child Health Insurance Program (SCHIP). *Pediatrics*. 1998;101:944–948

American Academy of Pediatrics Committee on Child Health Financing. Scope of health care benefits for newborns, infants, children, adolescents, and young adults through age 21 years. *Pediatrics*. 1997; 100:1040–1041

American Academy of Pediatrics Committee on Child Health Financing and Committee on State Government Affairs. Medicaid principles and sample legislative language. Medicaid model bill. Elk Grove Village, IL: American Academy of Pediatrics; June 1997

American Academy of Pediatrics Project Advisory Committee for the Medical Home Program for Children with Special Needs, Committee on Child Health Financing, and Committee on Children with Disabilities. *Managed Care and Children with Special Health Care Needs*. Elk Grove Village, IL: American Academy of Pediatrics; 1997

Behrman RE, ed. Children and managed health care. *Future Child*. Summer/Fall 1998;8(theme issue):4–160

Gellert GA. *Confronting Violence: Answers to Questions about the Epidemic Destroying America's Homes and Communities.* Boulder, CO: Westview Press; 1997

Sibbald WJ, Massaro TA, eds. *The Business of Critical Care: A Textbook for Clinicians Who Manage Special Care Units.* Armonk, NY: Future Publishing Co.; 1996

Resources

AAP: (1) Strategies for Managed Care: An Update from the Committee on Child Health Financing (newsletter). Emergency medical services for children and managed care, April 1997; (2) How to Use Your Managed Care Plan Effectively: Questions and Answers for Families with Children (brochure).

EMSC National Resource Center: (1) When Your Child Needs Help in a Hurry: A Parent's Guide to Selecting a Health Plan, reference number 0612; (2) Managed Care and EMSC: A Practical Guide to Resources in Managed Care, reference number 0571; (3) Caring for Kids in a Managed Care Environment (fact sheet), reference number 0583.

Surgery in the Office

Key Points for Surgical Procedures in the Office

1. Do not perform procedures that require deep sedation.
2. Prepare the patient and family for the procedure.
3. Ensure that needed supplies are available before the procedure.
4. Adhere to universal precautions.

Introduction

A number of minor surgical procedures can be performed safely and effectively in the pediatrician's office. Performing minor surgical procedures in the office allows the child to remain in a familiar environment and spares the parents the anxiety of making an additional trip to another facility. With some planning and a little experience, one can learn to do these procedures quickly and with little discomfort to the child.

This chapter reviews (1) the basic principles of performing minor surgical procedures in the office and (2) the minor surgical procedures that are best suited for the office setting.

General Principles

Several basic guidelines for office procedures are:

1. *Limit the procedures to those that can be done safely and effectively.*

   Safety should be the single most important consideration when deciding if a procedure is appropriate for the office. Safety implies the ability to handle potential complications of the procedure. An effectively done procedure can be done quickly, successfully, and with minimal discomfort to the child. Pharmacologic adjuncts to minimize pain and provide sedation can be used in the office setting. Chapter 6 describes the principles of analgesia and sedation appropriate for the office.

   The decision to perform a procedure on any child must be determined on a case-by-case basis. Factors in the decision include the time necessary for the procedure, the need for conscious or deep sedation, the availability of proper instruments or equipment, and the experience and skill of the physician.

2. *Do not attempt procedures that require deep sedation or general anesthesia.*

   Procedures requiring either general anesthesia or deep sedation should not be performed in most offices. These procedures should be done only at facilities that have the resources to properly monitor children during and after procedures and to remedy anesthetic complications.

3. *Prepare the patient and family for the procedure.*

   Preparing the child and family for the procedure increases the chance that the procedure will go smoothly. The procedure should be explained to both the child and the parents. Specifically, the parents need to understand why the procedure is needed, why the child might need to be restrained, and what will be done to minimize discomfort. Potential complications also need to be explained. Parental presence during a procedure often reduces stress for the child and the parent. At times, parents may be unable or may not wish to observe the procedure. Each situation is different and must be evaluated prior to initiation of the surgical procedure.

4. *Ensure that the needed supplies are available prior to beginning the procedure.*

   Delay in completion of a procedure is often due to not having the appropriate staffing and necessary equipment assembled before starting. Select and arrange supplies for use before the child is brought into the area. Prepared kits, trays, or carts for the most common procedure (eg, lacerations and abscesses) can greatly simplify preparation. Disposable instruments are inexpensive and dispense with the need for resterilization.

5. *Adhere to the Centers for Disease Control and Prevention (CDC) recommendations regarding universal precautions to minimize exposure risks during the procedure.*

   CDC recommendations for universal precautions may be obtained from Web site http://www.cdc.gov.

Anesthesia for Minor Surgical Procedures

Although some minor surgical procedures require only gentle reassurance and carefully chosen words, most procedures in children will require some sort of restraint, analgesia, or sedation. Restraining a child properly for a painful procedure can reduce pain, as well as reduce the amount of time that it takes to perform a procedure and increase the likelihood of success. Anxiolytics, analgesics, and sedating agents can be used alone or in combination with restraint to perform the procedure (see Chapter 6).

There are several other options for reducing the amount of discomfort that a child will experience during minor procedures. These options include the use of topical anesthetics such as TAC (containing tetracaine, adrenaline, and cocaine) and EMLA cream (containing lidocaine and prilocaine) and locally injected anesthetics (eg, lidocaine, Bupivacaine); see Chapter 6.

Regional Anesthesia

Regional anesthesia is an effective method for decreasing the pain associated with a procedure. A regional anesthetic provides anesthesia in the distribution of the nerve blocked. Probably the most valuable regional block for the office practitioner is the digital block (see Section 2.3 of Table 11). The skin overlying the nerve to be blocked is anesthestized and then lidocaine (5 mg/kg) is infiltrated around the nerve in the same manner as it is for local anesthesia.

See Table 11 on the following pages for a list of minor surgical procedures that can be done in the office.

Table 11.

Minor Surgical Procedures That Can Be Done in the Office

1.0 Restraining a child
2.0 Anesthetic procedures
   2.1 Direct infiltration of a wound with local anesthesia
   2.2 Field block
   2.3 Digital nerve block
3.0 Wound closure
4.0 Incision and drainage of an abscess
5.0 Procedures concerning the eye
   5.1 Eversion of the eyelids
   5.2 Irrigation of the conjunctiva
   5.3 Eyelid retraction
   5.4 Conjunctival foreign body removal
6.0 Procedures concerning the ears
   6.1 Removal of a foreign body from the ear
7.0 Procedures concerning the nose
   7.1 Removal of a nasal foreign body
8.0 Orthopedic procedures
   8.1 Splinting of musculoskeletal injuries
      8.1.1 Finger splints
      8.1.2 Long arm posterior splint
      8.1.3 Posterior ankle splint
      8.1.4 Long leg posterior splint
      8.1.5 Application of a figure-of-eight harness
      8.1.6 Arm sling
   8.2 Reduction of nursemaid's elbow
9.0 Miscellaneous procedures
   9.1 Removal of rings
   9.2 Removal of fish hooks
   9.3 Drainage of a subungual hematoma
   9.4 Incision and drainage of a paronychia
   9.5 Removal of a subungual splinter
10.0 Care of minor burns
11.0 Care of minor animal bites
12.0 Removal of a hair tourniquet from a digit

The following list of procedures includes common examples but is not meant to be exhaustive. Several comprehensive textbooks on pediatric procedures are listed in the Resources section at the end of this chapter.

1.0 Restraining a Child

Indications
- All procedures in which children will be unmanageable

Potential Complications
- Mistrust (if not discussed truthfully)
- Bruising (rare)
- Respiratory or airway compromise from improperly applied restraints

Supplies
- Papoose or mummy wrap

Method
- Explain the procedure to the family and child.
- *Papoose.* Place the child supine on the papoose and expose the body area necessary for treatment. Wrap the child with the Velcro straps beginning with the midabdominal restraints.
- *Mummy wrap.* Fold a sheet lengthwise such that the width is equal to the distance from the patient's axilla to just below the symphysis pubis. Place the sheet across the treatment table. Place the patient supine across the sheet, leaving approximately one-third the length of the sheet on one side and two-thirds on the opposite side. Bring both sides of the sheet anterior to the arms. Wrap the remaining long length of the sheet around the trunk and upper extremities until the end is reached.
- See Figures 2 through 5 for alternative methods of restraint.

Refer
- Refer children when the procedure cannot be accomplished with simple restraint alone or in combination with simple analgesics, anxiolytics, or sedation.

continued

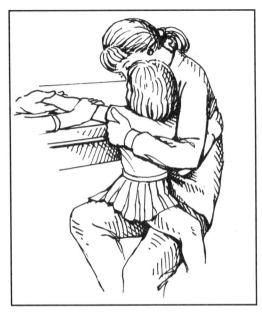

Fig 2. Immobilization for procedures can be safely accomplished by having the child sit facing the parent, encircled in a hug. Sitting up gives the child a sense of control and mastery. The child may watch the procedure if he or she wishes.

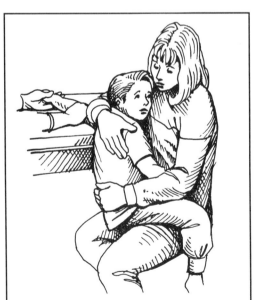

Fig 3. In the sitting position, the child can choose to look away.

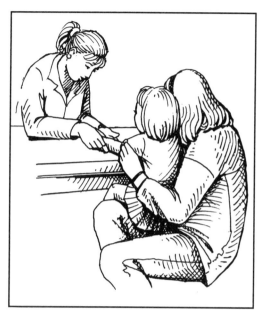

Fig 4. If the child cannot straddle the parent, because of injury or surgery, he or she can be positioned across the parent's knee.

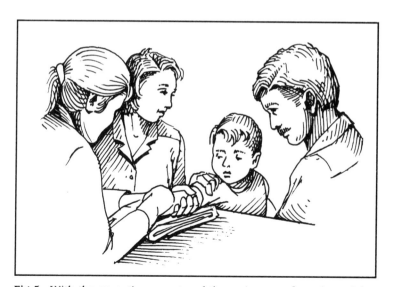

Fig 5. With the parent's support and the assistance of another adult to immobilize the limb, even a 2-year-old child can cooperate with procedures.

continued

2.1 Direct Infiltration of a Wound With Local Anesthesia

Indications
- Anesthesia for laceration repair

Potential Complications
- Bleeding
- Infection
- Intravascular injection resulting in seizures and cardiac arrest

Supplies
- Povidone-iodine solution
- 5-ml syringe
- Lidocaine (1% solution)
- Maximum dose 5 mg/kg (0.5 cc/kg of 1% solution)
- 26–30-gauge needle

Caution
- Avoid intravascular injections by aspirating prior to injection.
- Do not use lidocaine with epinephrine in end-arterial locations (fingers, toes, penis, nose, and earlobe).

Procedure
- Examine the injured area for deficits in blood supply, sensation, and motor function prior to injecting the anesthetic.
- Immobilize the child (see Section 1.0).
- Clean the area with povidone-iodine solution.
- Inject the anesthetic through the subcutaneous tissue exposed by the laceration by using a small-gauge needle. Begin the injection proximally to block nerve that supplies the more distal part of the wound.
- Wait 5 minutes for the anesthetic effect.

Refer
- Large wounds for which the dose of lidocaine required for the procedure would exceed the toxic dose.

2.2 Field Block

Indications
- Local anesthesia for procedures in areas of inflammation or infection or in areas where there is a benefit from preserving wound architecture.

Complications
- Bleeding
- Infection
- Intravascular injection resulting in seizures and cardiac arrest

Supplies
- Povidone-iodine solution
- 5-ml syringe
- Lidocaine (1% solution)
  Maximum dose 5 mg/kg (0.5 cc/kg of 1% solution)
- 26–30-gauge needle
- Biologics for tetanus prophylaxis

Procedure
- Examine the injured area for deficits in blood supply, sensation, and motor function prior to injecting the anesthetic.
- Immobilize the child (see Section 1.0).
- Clean the area with povidone-iodine solution.
- Anesthetize the area by using TAC or locally injected lidocaine. Field blocks utilize the same technique as that of direct wound infiltration, but the subdermis is entered through intact skin to prevent carrying debris or bacteria into uncontaminated tissues.
- Wait 5 to at least 25 minutes for the anesthesia to take effect.
- Test the area for anesthetic response.

2.3 Digital Nerve Block

Indications
- Anesthesia for procedures concerning the distal two-thirds of fingers and toes

Potential Complications
- Bleeding
- Infection

Caution
- Do not use lidocaine with epinephrine for digital blocks.

Supplies
- Povidone-iodine solution
- 5-ml syringe

continued

- Lidocaine (1% solution)
  Maximum dose 5 mg/kg (0.5 cc/kg of 1% solution)
- 26–30-gauge needle

Procedure

- Restrain the patient.
- Assess the digit for blood supply, sensation, and motor function before injecting the anesthetic agent.
- Clean the entire digit with povidone-iodine solution.
- Block the digital nerves at the level of the metacarpophalangeal joint. Inject both the medial and the lateral aspects of the proximal phalanx at the level of the web space. The digital nerves lie just superficial to the periosteum. The best way to ensure that the nerves are infiltrated is to advance the needle until it hits the bone. Prior to injection, the syringe should be aspirated to prevent an intravascular injection.
- Allow 5 minutes for the block to take effect.

Refer

Large and complicated wounds that require specialized care and wounds for which the dose of lidocaine would exceed the toxic dose

3.0 Wound Closure

Indications

- Lacerations

Complications

- Wound infection
- Scar formation

Caution

- Skin and mucous membrane trauma should be treated as dirty wounds with the potential for tetanus infection.

Supplies

- Povidone-iodine solution
- 5-ml syringe
- Lidocaine (1% solution)
  Maximum dose 5 mg/kg (0.5 cc/kg of 1% solution)
- 26–30-gauge needle
- Irrigation solution (normal saline)

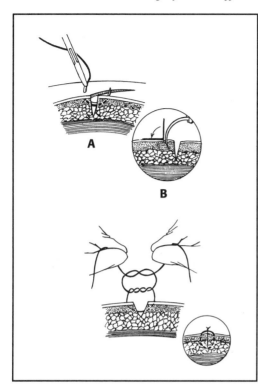

Fig 6. *(Top)* (A) The needle should enter the skin at a 90-degree angle. It should be inserted in a manner that allows it to follow a circular course. (B) For small wounds, the tip should become visible on the side of the wound opposite the entry site. *(Bottom)* The surgeon's knot, a double first throw followed by a single second throw, will help to maintain the integrity of the suture as it is tied.

- Needle holder
- Forceps
- Assortment of nylon sutures (4-0, 5-0, and 6-0)
- Sterile drapes
- Biologics for tetanus prophylaxis

Procedure

- Clean the wound and the surrounding area with povidone-iodine solution.
- Anesthetize the area to be sutured by using either TAC or locally injected lidocaine.
- Irrigate the wound with copious amounts of saline solution under pressure. A splash guard attached to a 35-ml syringe will create the needed pressure.
- Select the type and size of suture. The size of suture used is based on the site of the laceration. In general, 4.0 nylon suture is a good choice for most lacerations in children. Lacerations on the face should be repaired with a smaller suture (eg, 6.0 nylon).

continued

- Apply a dry dressing.
- Most sutures can be removed at 7 days, unless they are on the face, in which case they should be removed at 3–5 days (to prevent scarring), or in sites of tension, in which case they should remain in place for a longer period.
- Some lacerations can be closed with tissue adhesive products. Become familiar with the indications for their use and the procedure for application before using these products.

Refer

- Lacerations in cosmetic areas, wounds under high tension, and those that may require undermining or multiple layers of closure
- Lacerations where a foreign body is suspected or those that potentially implicate a joint, fracture, nerve, or tendon
- Puncture wounds that are deep and that may affect underlying structures such as nerves, vessels, tendons, and so forth

4.0 Incision and Drainage of an Abscess (Figure 7)

Indications

- Collection of pus that is not draining or adequately draining. An abscess should be drained when a fluctuant area is present. Once an abscess is present, warm soaks and antibiotics will not be effective. If there is a question of whether pus is present, the swelling can be aspirated with a needle and syringe.

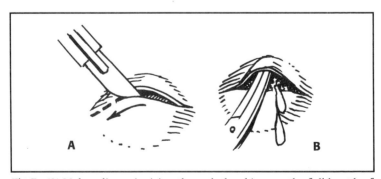

Fig 7. (A) Make a linear incision through the skin over the full length of the abscess cavity. Pay careful attention to avoid adjacent neurovascular structures. (B) Explore and drain the abscess cavity with a hemostat.

Potential Complications
- Bleeding
- Injuries to underlying structures
- Scar formation

Supplies
- Povidone-iodine solution
- Sterile drapes
- Lidocaine (1% solution)
- Syringes and needles (18–26 gauge)
- Number 11 scalpel blade
- Hemostat
- Iodoform gauze
- Dressing material

Method
- Clean the area with povidone-iodine solution.
- Administer a local anesthetic.
- Incise the abscess at the site of maximal fluctuance by using a number 11 scalpel blade.
- Pack with iodoform gauze. Leave a tail of gauze hanging from the wound to facilitate later removal. The purpose of packing the wound is to ensure that the skin remains open, allowing continued drainage from the wound, and to control bleeding.
- Apply a dry dressing and inform the parents that the abscess will continue to drain.
- Have the child return in 24–48 hours, at which time the drain is removed.
- Antibiotics are reserved for those patients who have surrounding cellulitis or lymphangitis.
- Consider the use of antibiotics for abscesses of the face, hand, and perineum.

Refer
- Facial abscesses
- Abscesses overlying vital structures (ie, large blood vessels)
- Perianal and perirectal abscesses
- Recurrent abscesses
- Abscesses in immunocompromised hosts

continued

5.1 Eversion of the Eyelids (Figure 8)

Indications

- Identification of a foreign body or infection
- Removal of a foreign body

Potential Complications

- Contusion (rare)
- Conjunctival abrasions
- Corneal abrasions

Supplies

- Cotton swab

Procedure

- Restrain the child.
- Upper lid: Grasp the eyelash and distal upper lid between the index finger and thumb. Ask the child to look downward if he or

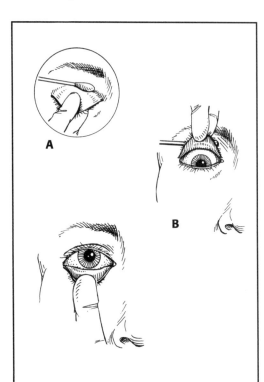

Fig 8. *(Top)* Eversion of upper eyelid: (A) place a cotton swab on the upper lid at the tarsal margin; (B) pull the swab downward as the eyelid is pulled upward to evert the lid. *(Bottom)* Eversion of lower eyelid.

she will cooperate. Draw the eyelid downward while applying
pressure to the superior tarsal plate with a cotton swab.
- Lower lid: Place a thumb or finger at the base of the lower lid and
gently retract it in a downward direction while the child is looking
upward.

5.2 Irrigation of the Conjunctiva (Figure 9)

Indications

- Presence of a caustic substance or foreign body on the cornea or
conjunctiva
- Begin irrigation as soon as possible to prevent complications and
eye damage.

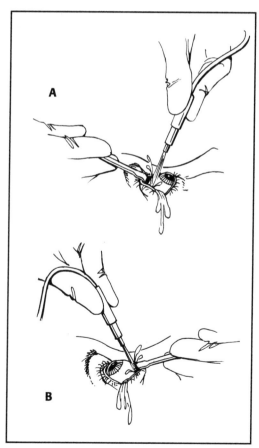

Fig 9. Irrigation of the eye. Direction of stream of saline in the (A) upper fornix and (B) lower fornix.

continued

Complications

- Conjunctivitis
- Subconjunctival hemorrhage or corneal abrasion (rare)

Supplies

- Normal saline intravenous fluid
- Intravenous tubing
- Gauze

Procedure

- Position the child supine over a large receptacle.
- Instill several drops of a topical anesthetic for ophthalmologic use.
- Hold the eye open by using gauze.
- Stream the fluid rapidly into the conjunctival sac.
- For caustic substances, irrigate immediately. For acid exposure, use at least 1 liter. For an alkali or unknown substance, use at least 2 liters. (This irrigation generally takes about 20 minutes.)

Refer

- For consultation with a poison-control center or ophthalmologist
- Pupil or iris irregularity
- Vision worse than baseline

5.3 Eyelid Retraction (Figure 10)

Indications

- Examination of the eye for suspected foreign bodies and for irrigation after chemical or toxic exposure. If ruptured globe is suspected, patch the eye and refer for ophthalmologic evaluation.
- Removal of a foreign body

Potential Complications

- Contusion of the lid
- Contusion of the globe
- Rupture or perforation of the globe
- Corneal abrasion

Supplies

- Topical anesthetic
- Eye speculum (Desmarres retractor or a simple metal paper clip fashioned into the appropriate shape)

Procedure

- Restrain the child.
- Place a drop of topical anesthetic in the bulbar conjunctiva.
- Slip the blade of the speculum under the lid margin and exert the traction upward or downward as indicated, as well as away from the globe.

Refer

- Suspected eye injuries
- Foreign bodies not easily removed
- Pupil or iris irregularity
- Vision worse than baseline

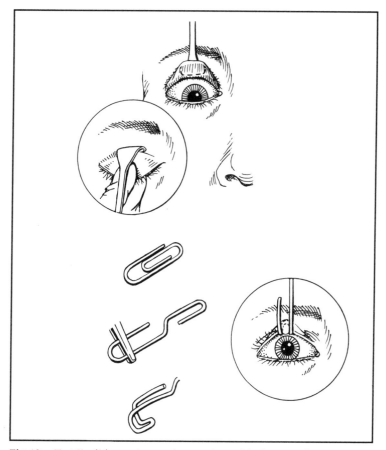

Fig 10. *(Top)* Eyelid eversion and retraction with the use of a Desmarres retractor. *(Bottom)* Standard paper clip fashioned into a lid retractor

continued

6.1 Removal of a Foreign Body From the Ear

Indications
• Presence of a foreign body in the ear

Potential Complications
• Laceration of the auditory canal wall (often unavoidable)
• Perforation of the tympanic membrane
• Ossicular disruption

Supplies
• Otoscope
• 50-ml syringe for irrigation
• Plastic vascular catheter
• Curette
• Alligator and bayonet forceps
• Water pick
• Suction device for foreign body removal
• Superglue adhesive

Procedure
• If not cooperative, the child will need to be restrained.
• Visualize the foreign body with the speculum. Assess whether the foreign body can be easily removed.
• Remove the foreign body. Removal can be done by using one of several techniques.
1. *Irrigation.* Use a 50-cc syringe attached to a flexible intravenous catheter tip. Irrigate the canal by injecting a constant stream of water at body temperature. Do not use this method if the object is subject to expansion from absorbing water.
2. *Curette.* Advance the curette beyond the foreign body and slowly withdraw the curette and object.
3. *Forceps.* Use direct vision to guide the forceps to the foreign body, with or without the use of an otoscope with speculum. Open the forceps just in front of the foreign body, grasp the object, and then slowly withdraw.
4. *Suctioning.* Use a specialized suctioning device that is manufactured for removal of foreign bodies (Schuknecht foreign body remover).
5. *Superglue.* Some foreign bodies can be removed by using superglue applied to a wooden applicator or similar object. Place glue-coated applicator on the foreign body and allow it to bond to the

object. Note that most commercially available glues will not bond to plastic objects. Avoid inadvertent contact with tissue surfaces.
• Visualize the ear drum and document its condition.

Refer

• Foreign bodies not easily visualized or those not easily removed on the first attempt

7.1 Removal of a Nasal Foreign Body (Figure 11)

Indications

• Presence of a nasal foreign body

Potential Complications

• Mucosal laceration
• Epistaxis
• Rhinosinusitis
• Aspiration of foreign body
• Incomplete removal of foreign body

Supplies

• Nasal speculum
• Light source (head light or directed light source)
• Suction
• Hook

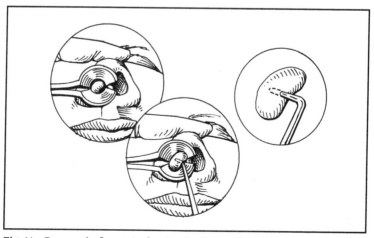

Fig 11. Removal of certain foreign bodies such as beans or beads may be facilitated by using a right-angle pick.

continued

- Alligator and bayonet forceps
- Vasoconstrictor nasal spray

Procedure

Several methods can be employed for the removal of a nasal foreign body.

- Restrain the child in the supine position. The patient must be kept still to prevent injury to the nasal mucosa during the procedure.
- Visualize the foreign body. The objects most amenable to removal in the office are those in the external part of the nares.
- Attempt removal by occluding the nonobstructed nares and having the parent forcibly blow into the child's mouth. Alternatively, a bag-valve-mask may be used by placing the mask over the child's mouth and delivering high-pressure ventilation. Use a large reservoir bag for this procedure (at least 750 ml).
- Attempt to extract the foreign body with suction, hook, or alligator forceps as determined by the size, nature, and position of the object.
- Avoid pushing the object into the posterior nasopharynx because it may be aspirated.

Refer

- Foreign bodies of the nose that are not easily visualized
- Objects that have been present for more than several days
- Objects not easily removed on the first attempt

8.1. Splinting of Musculoskeletal Injuries

8.1.2 Long Arm Posterior Splint (Figure 12)

Indications

Immobilization of elbow injuries and suspected fractures of the radius and ulna

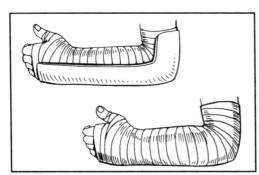

Fig 12. The long-arm posterior splint may be used to immobilize proximal forearm and elbow injuries.

Potential Complications

- Pressure injury (vascular compromise)

Supplies

- Cotton bandage (Webril)
- Plaster slab or ready-made plaster splint
- Elastic wrap (Ace)
- Sling

Procedure

- Expose the child's arm.
- Flex the elbow to 90 degrees.
- Apply a Webril bandage from the wrist to the shoulder.
- Apply the plaster splint to the posterior aspect of the joint.
- Apply an elastic wrap to hold the plaster in place.
- Apply a sling.

Refer

- Suspected fractures, dislocations, and ligament injuries

8.1.3. Posterior Ankle Splint (Figure 13)

Indications

- Immobilization of ankle sprains and fractures of the foot, ankle, and distal fibula

Potential Complications

- Pressure injury (vascular compromise)

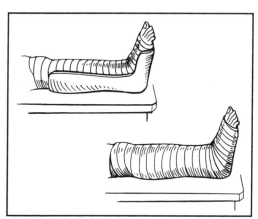

Fig 13. The posterior ankle splint may be used to immobilize ankle sprains and fractures of the foot, ankle, and distal fibula.

continued

Supplies

- Cotton bandage (Webril)
- Plaster slab or ready-made plaster splint
- Elastic wrap (Ace)

Procedure

- Expose the child's foot and ankle.
- Flex the ankle to 90 degrees.
- Apply a Webril bandage from the toes to just below the knee.
- Apply the plaster splint to the posterior aspect of the joint.
- Apply an elastic wrap to hold the plaster in place.

Refer

- Suspected fractures, dislocations, and ligament injuries

8.1.4 Long Leg Posterior Splint (Figure 14)

Indications

- Immobilization of suspected knee injuries and fractures of the tibia and fibula

Potential Complications

- Pressure injury (vascular compromise)

Supplies

- Cotton bandage (Webril)
- Plaster slab or ready-made plaster splint
- Elastic wrap (Ace)

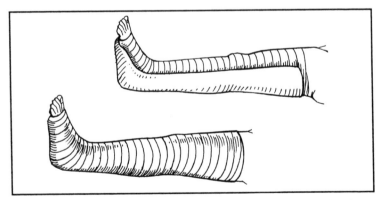

Fig 14. The long-leg posterior splint may be used to immobilize knee injuries and fractures of the tibia and fibula.

Procedure

- Expose the child's leg, foot, and ankle.
- Flex the ankle to 90 degrees and the knee to 45 degrees.
- Apply a Webril bandage from the ankle to the area just below the gluteal fold.
- Apply the plaster splint to the posterior aspect of the joint.
- Apply an elastic wrap to hold the plaster in place.

Refer

- Suspected fractures, dislocations, and ligament injuries

8.1.5 Application of a Figure-of-eight Harness (Figure 15)

Indications

- Midshaft clavicular fracture

Complications

- Pressure sore (applied too tight)

Supplies

- Figure-of-eight harness

Procedure

- Obtain a radiogram to confirm the presence and location of the fracture.

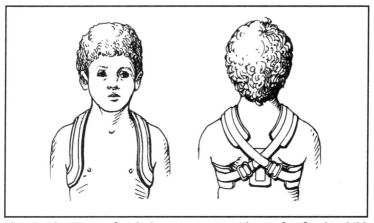

Fig 15. The Figure-of-eight harness can provide comfort for the child with a clavicle fracture. If the a harness is unavailable, a sling may be used in its place.

continued

- Choose the appropriate-sized harness.
- Apply the harness while the child is standing. The harness should fit snugly, and the shoulders should be straight. Tighten the straps as necessary.
- Before the parents leave the office, teach them how to reapply the harness.
- Instruct the patient to wear the harness for 3 weeks (except while bathing).

8.2 Reduction of Nursemaid's Elbow (Figures 16 and 17)

Indications

- Suspected radial head subluxation (nursemaid's elbow).
  This injury is common in the toddler age group. The injury results from excessive axial traction placed across the elbow joint.

Potential Complications

- Vascular or musculoskeletal trauma if the maneuver is performed on a child with a fracture

Procedure

- Establish the diagnosis. Obtain a clear history of the injury. The affected arm is generally held at the child's side, slightly flexed at the elbow in pronation. Point tenderness along the length of the arm or shoulder suggests a fracture.
- Explain the planned procedure to the parents.
- Grasp the palm of the child's hand as if to shake it. Encircle the elbow with the other hand with the thumb over the annular ligament of the radius. Gently supinate the palm of the hand and in a continuous motion flex the elbow to the shoulder. During the flexion maneuver, the physician feels a "pop" with the thumb that lies over the radial head. Hyperpronation is an alternate maneuver.
- The child should use the arm freely and without pain within a few minutes.
- Radiograms are indicated only if a fracture is suspected or if reduction is unsuccessful after two or three attempts.

Refer

- When this maneuver does not improve the child's symptoms or there is a suspected fracture

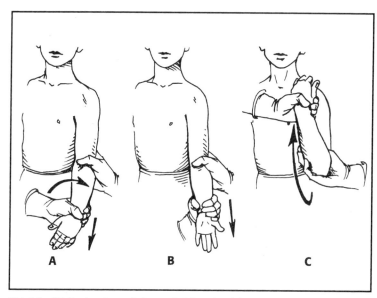

Fig 16. (A) Reduction of the radial head subluxation begins with axial traction applied to the forearm with the wrist adducted to the ulnar side. Pressure is also applied directly over the radial head at the level of the antecubital fossa. (B) The forearm is supinated while axial traction and pressure are maintained over the radial head. (C) The forearm is then flexed while supination and pressure are maintained over the radial head.

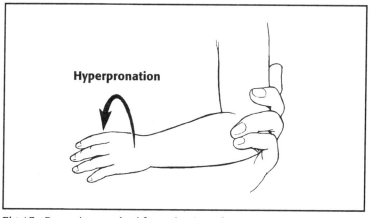

Fig 17. Pronation method for reduction of nursemaid's elbow, demonstrating hyperpronation at the wrist.

continued

9.1 Removal of Rings (Figure 18)

Indications

• Unremovable rings

Potential Complications

• Trauma to digit
• Vascular compromise

Supplies

• Ring cutter
• String (3.0 silk suture)
• Ice water

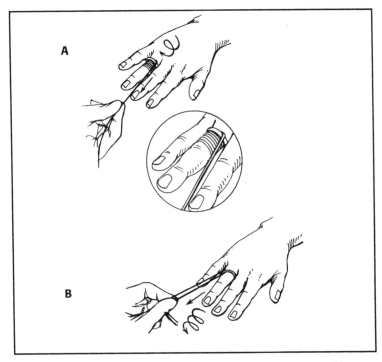

Fig 18. *(Top)* (A) String compression method. Whenever possible, move ring to most proximal aspect of the digit before wrapping suture around the finger. The use of a digital block and a generous amount of lubricant will contribute to a successful outcome. *(Bottom)* (B) String pull method. Using a continuous circular motion, pull the suture around the finger.

Procedure

- Make an assessment of the value of the ring. If the ring is of no value, the simplest method of removing the ring is to use a ring cutter. The ring cutter divides the ring allowing separation from the finger.
- When a ring cutter is not available or there is a strong desire to preserve the ring, several other methods can be used.
1. *String compression method.* Wrap a 3.0 silk suture around the finger, starting at the distal edge of the ring. Continue to wrap the string tightly until it covers the proximal interphalangeal joint. Pull the ring over the wrapped suture and off the finger.
2. *String pull.* Use a string or heavy suture. Place one end of the string under the ring. Pull the string thorough. Place a small amount of lubricating ointment at the distal end of the ring. Pull the suture in a circular motion.
3. *Ice water.* Soak the hand in cold water. Soap the finger and twist the ring off.

Refer

- Digits if there may be vascular compromise

9.2 Removal of Fishhooks (Figure 19)

Indications

- Embedded fishhook in the skin

Potential Complications

- Tissue damage
- Risk of infection

Supplies

- Povidone-iodine solution
- 5-ml syringe (25- or 27-gauge needle)
- Lidocaine (1% solution)
- Needle holders
- Number 11 scalpel blade
- Biologics for tetanus prophylaxis

Procedure

- Prepare the skin with povidone-iodine solution.
- Anesthetize the affected area with lidocaine (1% solution).
- Cut the barb by grasping the fishhook with needle holders and

continued

advancing the hook out through the skin in the curve of the hook. Cut the barb off with a wire cutter. Withdraw the remaining hook along the original path of entry. This method may not work when the fishhook is deeply embedded.

- Apply a dry dressing.
- Assess tetanus immunization status and give appropriate biologics as indicated.

Refer

- Deeply embedded fishhooks
- Fishhooks embedded in the eye

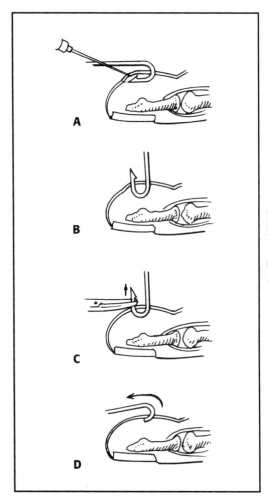

Fig 19. Cutting off a hook barb. This technique is ideal for smaller or superficially located hooks.

9.3 Drainage of a Subjungual Hematoma (Figure 20)

Indications

• Collection of blood under pressure beneath the nail bed

Potential Complications

• Bleeding
• Infection

Supplies

• Povidone-iodine solution
• Electrocautery unit or heated paper clip to burn a hole in the nail

Procedure

• Restrain the child's hand.
• Burn a hole in the nail by using the electrocautery unit or the heated paper clip. Several holes should be made to ensure adequate drainage.
• Instruct the patient to keep the area clean, and inform him or her that the nail may be lost.

Refer

• Suspected nail-bed injury or distal phalanx fracture

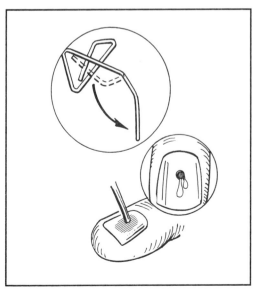

Fig 20. Drainage of subungual hematoma can be accomplished either by a portable cautery device or by the use of a heated paper clip.

continued

9.4 Incision and Drainage of a Paranychia (Figure 21)

Indications

- Failure of a paronychia to respond to medical management (soaks and antibiotics) with presence of pus

Potential Complications

- Bleeding
- Scar formation

Supplies

- Povidone-iodine solution
- Lidocaine (1% solution)
- Number 11 scalpel blade
- Syringes and needles (21–26 gauge)
- Scissors and forceps
- Sterile nonstick dressings

Procedure

- Clean the digit with povidone-iodine solution.
- Administer a digital block.
- Incise the paronychia by using a number 11 scalpel blade held parallel to the nail bed. A small strip of nail may need to be removed, depending on the size of the paronychia.
- Instruct the patient to soak the digit several times a day.

Refer

- Recurrent paronychias that may need nail removal if you are unfamiliar with the technique or the infection is deep

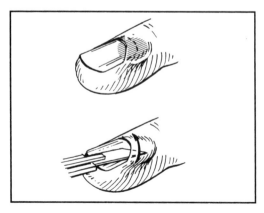

Fig 21. Method for drainage of a simple paronychia.

9.5 Removal of a Subungual Splinter (Figure 22)

Indications

- Painful subungual splinter
- To prevent infection or a foreign body reaction to the splinter in the nail bed

Potential Complications

- Bleeding

Supplies

- Povidone-iodine solution
- Number 11 scalpel blade
- Small forceps
- Biologics for tetanus prophylaxis

Procedure

- Restrain the child's hand.
- Use a number 11 scalpel blade to scrape the nail down to the level of the nail bed. Continue this process until the splinter is exposed and can be grasped with a small forceps. Large splinters may require prolonged scraping and are best removed under a digital block.

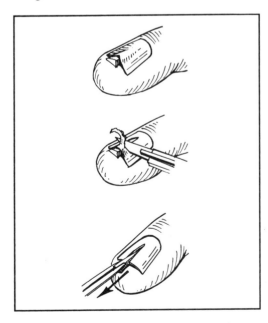

Fig 22. *(Top)* Use a scalpel to remove a small wedge of nail overlying the splinter. *(Bottom)* Use a forceps to remove the foreign body.

continued

- Alternatively, pass a needle under the nail beneath the splinter. Trap the splinter between the needle and nail and slide out.
- Soak the finger in warm povidone-iodine solution several times a day to decrease the chance of infection.
- Assess the tetanus immunization status of the patient and give appropriate tetanus prophylaxis.

Refer
- When there is significant injury to the nail bed

10.0 Care of Minor Burns

Indications
- Superficial partial thickness burns
- Surface area less that 5% of the total body surface area of the child
- Burns that **do not** affect the face, hands, feet, or any intertrigenous area (perineum, neck, axillae)

Complications
- Infection
- Scarring

Supplies
- Normal saline
- Sterile scissors and forceps
- Topical antibiotic cream (silver sulfadiazine, mupirocin, or bacitracin)
- Biologics for tetanus prophylaxis

Procedure
- Cleanse the burn area with normal saline.
- Determine the size and severity of the burn.
- Debride all necrotic tissue.
- Blister removal is determined by the size, location, and practice standard of the community.
- Apply a topical antibiotic cream. Do not use silver-containing materials on the face or any area where discoloration may not be desirable.
- Assess tetanus immunization status and give prophylaxis as appropriate.

Refer

- All large burns (greater than 5% of total body surface area)
- All deep partial-thickness and full-thickness burns
- All burns to the face, hands, feet, perineum, and intertriginous areas.

11.0 Care of Animal Bites

- Various animals may bite children. Dog and cat bites are the most common animal bites.

Indications

- Small superficial uncomplicated wounds

Complications

- Infection
- Rabies

Supplies

- Normal saline
- Sterile dressing
- Topical antibiotic cream
- Biologics for tetanus prophylaxis

Procedure

- Inspect the wound.
- Irrigate the wound profusely with normal saline.
- Apply topical antibiotic cream.
- Consider systemic antibiotics. The use of antibiotics will be determined by the type of animal bite, the site, and the extent of injury.

Refer

- Deep or extensive wounds to the face or hands
- Any deep wound
- Wounds where damage to underlying structures such as nerves, vessels, or tendons are affected

12.0 Removal of a Hair Tourniquet from a Digit

Indications

- Hair wrapped tightly around a digit

continued

Complications

- Tissue necrosis
- Infection
- Loss of digit

Supplies

- Forceps
- Scissors
- Number 11 scalpel blade
- Fine needle
- Good light source

Procedure

- Several methods can be used for the removal of a hair tourniquet. Use the method with which you are most familiar.
- Identify the hair tourniquet.
- Grasp the hair with a fine forceps.
- Cut the hair with a blade or scissors.

Alternate Method

- Identify the hair tourniquet.
- Insert the tip of a very fine needle (27–30 gauge) under the hair.
- Cut the hair by using the needle tip or a blade or scissors.

Refer

- Any area in which there is vascular compromise
- Digits with lacerations
- Unsuccessful removal of the tourniquet

••

All figures in this chapter are reprinted with permission from Walsh-Suskys M, Krug SE. Procedures in Infants and Children. *Philadelphia, PA; Saunders. Copyright 1997.*

Resources

Dieckmann RA, Fiser DH, Selbst SM. *Illustrated Textbook of Pediatric Emergency and Critical Care Procedures.* St. Louis, MO: Mosby; 1997

Henretig FM, King C. *Textbook of Pediatric Emergency Procedures.* Philadelphia, PA: Williams & Wilkins; 1997

Available On-line Resources

Key Points About the Internet

1. Many EMS-C- specific sites are available on the Internet.
2. Databases are available from the Internet to aid in planning.
3. Funding sources are available from the Internet.

Introduction

In the past decade, the Internet and the World Wide Web (WWW) have gone from the realm of research laboratories into the homes and offices of millions of people. The array and accessibility of resources on the Internet has increased dramatically in the past few years. The Internet and the WWW have developed into powerful tools for the healthcare provider. The "net" offers a rich multimedia format including video, sound, interactive instruction, and more. It affords the physician an opportunity to communicate with other physicians, organizations, and families in the "net" community. There are many well-developed Internet resources for EMS-C.

As with any new tool, there are unexpected uses and limitations. Efficient and judicious use of the Internet is essential to optimize effectiveness. Developing strategies for use and gaining experience quickly mitigates any initially overwhelming aspect of the Internet.

Information on the Internet must be inspected carefully for accuracy, objectivity, currency, and authority. A Web site may appear professionally produced and impressive, even when the information is biased or inaccurate. As a general rule, users should always answer the following questions when using information from a Web site:

1. Who is the author(s) of the site?
2. What is the source of the information? Does the site have listed references?
3. Is the information biased?
4. Is the information accurate? Can it be corroborated?
5. Is the Web site current? When was the last update?

Internet Basics

The Internet for all of its possibilities and seemingly endless complexity is at its heart simply an interconnection between computers. In the early days of the Internet, text was the only means of transferring information. The first components of the Internet, which are text based, such as GOPHER, are still in existence. As computer processor and modem speed increased, faster data transfer was possible, allowing the use of sound, video, and pictures. The use of this multimedia environment encouraged the explosive growth, and interconnections between computers grew.

Individual users, institutions, or organizations can construct a "site" that is accessible to any other computer. This site is located, or "hosted," on a host computer with connections to the Internet; it is through these connections that the site can be viewed. Internet service providers (ISPs), who serve as the middleman between the computer user and the Internet, provide the physical connection to the Internet. ISPs vary in the services offered. The larger ISPs (AOL, MSN, etc.) provide specialty services and programming for entertainment, financial, and other services. Some ISPs simply serve as a conduit to the Internet. When choosing an ISP, there are several important considerations to keep in mind:

1. Is the company stable and established? What is its reputation?
2. Access: Is it easy to dial in and get connected? A small ISP may not have enough access lines and you will get a busy signal when you try to connect.
3. Does the ISP offer the services that you need, such as electronic mail (e-mail), live communication (chat), and browsing?
4. Cost: Is there a flat fee for unlimited usage?
5. Support: Is 24-hour support available? Is there a help center?

Once you have logged onto the Internet, several basic services are available to most users. These services include browsing, e-mail and list servers, chat, and video exchange. Whether one has the ability to utilize all of these services depends on the service provider and the computer's capabilities.

World Wide Web Browsing

The terms World Wide Web and Internet are often used interchangeably. In truth, the WWW is a subsection of the Internet. The WWW consists of Web sites that are composed of text as well as pictures and may include audio and video. A Web browser is a program that allows Web sites to be accessed and information to be passed from the Web site to the computer user and, likewise, from the computer user to the Web site. There are some important facts about viewing the WWW through a Web browser.

- Each Web site and each page on a Web site has a unique site address. This site address allows a Web browser to return to that site quickly and efficiently.
- An individual Web site may have many levels and layers. Some Web sites can be very complex and require time for complete exploration.
- When you arrive at a Web site, you usually arrive at what is called a "home page." The home page is the first page of information presented to the computer user by the Web site and contains a "road map" of that particular Web site.
- On the home page, there are "hyperlinks." These hyperlinks are usually pictures or text that, when selected, will lead you to another page on that same Web site that contains specific information, as indicated by the picture or text on the home page.
- By selecting or clicking on the hyperlinks, you are able to "navigate" that specific Web site.
- Web sites vary greatly in regard to complexity, ease of use, and usefulness. Web sites may be interlinked between each other, and one Web site may lead to a completely different Web site that may have a subject similar to that of the original Web site.

Electronic Mail and List Servers

E-mail has developed into a fast and reliable means of communication throughout the world. To use e-mail, you type a message, address it to a specific person or organization, and "mail" the communication over the computer connection. E-mail can consist of text as well as attached files, which can include video, audio, or computer programs. The advantages of e-mail include speed, ease of use, and ability to send files. Concerns include matters of privacy and confidentiality. E-mail is *not* secure communication and may be erroneously addressed, delivered, or read by persons for whom it was not intended. E-mail may also not be protected by First Amendment rights at many organizations and institutions. Messages that contain information that is confidential or privileged should not be sent by e-mail.

List servers are a way for groups of people with a specific interest to send messages to a common address and then, from that address, the message is delivered to all subscribers. Lists are arranged by topics of interest; specific topics of discussion may vary according to the member's interest or according to the discussion "thread." A "thread" is a series of discussions about a specific topic within a list server. At times a "thread" may become so significant or permanent that it will become its own specific list server.

List servers are an effective means of communication between many people on a specific topic, and each list has its own rules. Some list servers will allow all messages, whereas many have specific criteria. Most list servers have a moderator to oversee the list topic development and maintain order if the discussions get too tangential or heated. There are two well-known sites that compile lists of list servers every week and are searchable by keyword: the Listz Directory (http://www.sparklist.com/) and the Lists of Lists (http://www.catalog.com/vivian/interest-group-search.html).

If there is not a Web site that addresses your interests, start your own site. Many educational institutions allow students and faculty to have individual list servers or Web sites. In addition, many companies will host a list server for a low monthly fee. A large list of list physicians with rates and more detailed information can be found at http://www.catalog.com/vivian/mailing-list-physicians.html.

Usenet News Groups

Usenet comprises news groups arranged by topic. A news group contains postings called articles that may be read by the newsgroups users. Replies to postings can be added to a news group and are available for all members to see. A news group differs from a mailing list in that messages are not sent to each individual subscriber; rather they are housed in one location available for browsing. A news group is the equivalent of an electronic bulletin board. There are two useful locators of usenet news groups: Deja News (http://www.dejanews.com) and Search for Groups (http://www.sunsite.unc.edu/usenet-i/search.html). These sites allow you to search for postings in news groups by keyword. These postings can then be reviewed and, if you are interested, you can join the news group and post a reply or an entirely new article.

Discussion (Chat) Groups

Chat groups consist of people who meet "live" in "real time" on the Internet. Chat sites are usually arranged by areas of interest, are convened at specific times, and may or may not have moderators or guests. Chat sites allow for real time communication in a text format between people. These sites allow for a rich and varied exchange of information among people throughout the world. Video chat sites are currently offered on the WWW; however, a video chat site requires both a camera to be hooked up to the user's computer and some special software. Some mailing lists such as PedTalk have scheduled chat sessions.

Searching the Internet

Effectively and efficiently searching the WWW is a valuable skill. The overwhelming amount of information on the WWW can be managed with a skillful search. A search engine is a Web site dedicated to searching the WWW for sites of interest to the computer user. Several large search engines on the Internet have strategies for searching the WWW. These sites allow a user to manage the seemingly infinite and daunting amount of information present on the WWW. Different Web sites vary in their search paradigms and methods; using one search engine consistently will enable you to become comfortable with searching the WWW and refining your searches. Often, if the search engine does not return a specific match that a user is seeking, visiting one of those Web sites that are returned will allow the user to link from a site of moderate interest to related sites that may be more pertinent. Search engines can be divided into two broad groups: subject catalogs and WWW search engines. Subject catalogs search the WWW for Web sites pertaining to the subject entered, whereas search engines look at the actual documents (Web pages) for occurrences of the keyword. You can see that searching for a common word with a WWW search engine will return an enormous list of Web pages.

Subject Catalogs

- *Yahoo!* (http://www.yahoo.com). Yahoo! is a powerful database that can be personalized by selecting My Yahoo!. Yahoo! also has a search engine for kids, Yahooligans (http://www.yahooligans.com). Searches are performed by keywords and Web sites.
- *Argus Clearinghouse* (http://www.clearinghouse.net/). This site allows for Boolean searches, search operators, and truncations. Results displayed include guide title, author name, keywords, and ratings.
- *Galaxy* (http://www.einet.net/). This site provides a topic list linking one page to the next. Searches also can be undertaken.

Search Engines

- *All in One Search* (http://www.albany.net/allinone/all1www.html). This engine provides one page access to all major search engines on the Web. It allows the user to link to many search engines easily and efficiently
- *Alta Vista* (http://www.altavista.digital.com/)
- *Excite!* (http://www.excite.com)
- *Lycos* (http://www.lycos.com)
- *Webcrawler* (http://www.webcrawler.com/)
- *Hotbot* (http://www.hotbot.com). This site merges numerous search engines into one and returns the result.

  Name, e-mail, and address or telephone number also can be used to search for individuals.

- *Four 11* (http://www.four11.com)
- *Who Where* (http://www.whowhere.com)
- *555-1212*.com (http://www555-1212.com)

Medical Search Engines

- *CLINIWEB* (http://www.ohsu.edu/cliniweb/search.html). A *very useful* site that allows you to enter a disease name or condition and returns pages that match your keyword.
- *Health A to Z* (http://www.healthatoz.com/). A large database that covers many health-related fields.

Emergency Medical Services for Children on the WWW

With the increase in use and sophistication of the WWW, the quality, type, and amount of information available has increased dramatically. The Internet offers those interested in EMS-C a vast array of resources in many areas, including but not limited to:

- Networking among the medical community and EMS-C physicians
- Interactive education
- Organizations
- Research
- Data sources
- Government resources

Networking

The Internet allows for effective communication between health-care service physicians and families. It is possible to join EMS-C-related list servers, news groups, and chat groups. If used effectively, this means of communication can be a rapid and effective tool for linking the EMS-C community.

Mailing Lists of Interest

- *Emergency Medical Services List.* The purpose of this list is to provide emergency medical services professionals and friends with an open forum in which to share experience, suggestions, and gripes about topics related to the EMS profession. To subscribe, send an e-mail to listproc2@ecnet.net, and, in the message body, type "subscribe emschat" and your full name.
- *Pediatric Emergency Medicine List.* PED-EM-List is an international forum for professionals interested in the emergency

care of children. To join the list, send an e-mail to list-serv@brownvm.brown.edu, and, in the message body, type "subscribe PED-EM-L" and your name.

- *Emergency Medical Services Educators List.* The EMS-EDU-L list is a moderated one, although it was not in the recent past. A moderated list means that messages will not be distributed until and unless they have been reviewed by the list owner(s). To subscribe, send a message to listserver@informaties. sunysb.edu, and, in the message body, type "subscribe ems-edu-1" and your full name.
- *International Pediatric Chat* (http://www.pedschat.org/). This is an Internet relay chat channel with an Internet interface for pediatricians and other child health professionals.
- *National Association of EMS Physicians List.* A list server maintained by NAEMSP. To subscribe, send an e-mail to list-serv@listserv.acns.nwu.edu, and, in the message body, type "subscribe ems-l".
- *PEDTALK.* A general pediatric discussion mailing list. To subscribe, send an e-mail to pedtalk-request@pcc.com, and, in the body, type "subscribe."
- *Pediatric Health.* This list is an electronic newsletter of timely tips and useful facts concerning the physical and mental health of infants, children, and adolescents. To subscribe, send an e-mail to schneider@mtwest.net with the word "subscribe." Leave the message body blank.
- *Child Health List.* The goals of child health are to provide up-to-date information about developments in evidence-based child health and to promote the practice of evidence-based medicine related to children. To subscribe, send an e-mail to listserv@cgnet.com containing the message "SUBSCRIBE CHILDHEALTH-CFOC."

General Medical Sites

- *Achoo* (http://www.achoo.com). Includes a searchable database, news group discussion, and many links to other sites.
- *Medway* (http://www.cc.emory.edu/whscl/medweb.html). Extensive links to many medical sites.
- *Doctors Guide to the Internet* (http://www.pslgroup.com/ Docguide.htm). One of the best sites on the web. Extensive

links to hospitals, databases, and organizations. A great site to explore.

- *Ped Info: An Index of Pediatric Internet* (http://www.uab.edu/ pedinfo/). This is an excellent general site that has Internet resources divided into pediatric forums, condition- or disease-specific information, and subspecialties in areas of study. There are also links to children's hospitals, educational sites, and pediatricians on-line, as well as government agencies and child-advocacy organizations. This is an excellent site to begin exploring the pediatric Internet.

- *Physicians Guide to the Internet* (http://www.webcom. com/pgi/).

- *Yahoo!* (http://www.yahoo.com/Health). Offers many subcategories by specialty and interest. Makes initial Web surfing very easy.

Education

Many Web sites exist on the Internet that have been created by organizations or persons who provide education in EMS-C. The host of educational opportunities on the WWW is truly astounding. There exist, available for downloading, movies of procedures from bronchoscopes to line placements to examination of patients. Heart sounds, EKGs, radiography files, and virtual patients can be accessed on the WWW. The educational opportunities are truly endless. Again, it is important to note that many Web sites are not peer reviewed, and it is important to assess the quality of information presented. Compared with privately published anecdotal sites, Web sites of major institutions name authors, list references, and provide for feedback and have made an effort to qualify their information. There are several well-developed and useful Web sites for education in EMS-C and pediatric emergency medicine.

- *Emergency Medicine and Primary Care Home Page* (http://www. embbs.com/). This is a well-developed Web site that is updated frequently and has a dedicated backing of experienced physicians. It includes:
  - Pediatric emergency medicine topics featuring in-depth radiology cases in pediatric emergency medicine
  - Computer tomography (CT) scan library
  - Medical photograph library

- Radiology library
- Pediatric advance life-support megacode simulator and interactive pediatric patient care simulation. This is an excellent run-through of the pediatric code with an interactive format, allowing the user to administer drugs, review the progress of the patient, and perform procedures in an interactive virtual environment.
- Electrocardiogram of the month and EKG file room
- Cases and photographs from the *Journal of the Society for Academic Emergency Medicine*
- Medical software showcase
- Emergency medical systems update with links to other EMS sites on the Web
- *Injury Control* (http://www.injurycontrol.com/icrin/). This is a large list of Internet resources related to the field of injury research and control. This well-developed Web site offers links to federal and state agencies, injury data and statistics, and specific resources on types of injuries.
  - *Injury-Free Coalition for Kids* (http://www.injuryfree.org).
  - *Hypertox* (http://www.ozemail.com.au/ ~ ouad/toxi0002.htm) Hypertox is an excellent resource for toxicology and offers a hypertext document that covers toxicology issues as well as specific toxidromes. It is an interactive learning format and can be downloaded from the Web site to a host computer.
- *MEDCONNECT* (http://www.medconnect.com/index.htm). This is an excellent site for interactive education, interactive jobs lines, access to Medline, and access to Health A to Z (search engine for health and medicine), and it allows for continuing medical education (CME) credits. Membership to this site is free of charge. However, there is a small charge for receiving CME credits. This site features:
  - Pediatric cases of the month
  - Developmental rounds
  - Pediatric EKG casebooks
  - Dilemmas in ambulatory pediatrics
  - Selected cases in toxicology
  - Pediatric News at Your Desktop: an on-line newsletter that features articles from various pediatric peer-review journals as well as a commentary. Overall, this is an excellent site

that also offers interactive job lines, meetings and conferences, and a managed-care forum.

- *Radiology Cases in Pediatric Emergency Medicine* (http://www. hawaii.edu/medicine/pediatrics/pemxray/pemxray.html). This site allows radiology cases in pediatric emergency medicine to be downloaded and placed on a host computer. Excellent-quality radiographs are available as well as case presentations accompanying each radiograph. This is a first-class site for learning about pediatric emergency radiology.
- *RX List: The Internet Drug Index* (http://www.rxlist.com/). This Web site gives drug information, including interactions and actions of medications. This site also allows unknown tablets to be identified by searching for their ID imprint codes. It is also possible to search by keyword through all the drug monologues.
- *The Virtual ER* (http://www.virtualer.com). This site offers emergency medicine tutorials, clinical and radiological images, and a medical library with search capabilities.
- *The Virtual Children's Hospital* (http://www.vch.vh.org). Developed by the Department of Radiology, University of Iowa College of Medicine, this site provides interactive pediatric resources, including on-line textbooks and other publications, radiographic teaching files, and case simulations.

Publications On-line

- *Academic Emergency Medicine* (http://www.hanleyandbelfus. com/journals/aem.html). The official journal of the Society for Academic Emergency Medicine.
- *Annals of Emergency Medicine* (http://www.mosby.com/ Mosby/Periodicals/Medical/AEM/em.html). The official journal of the American College of Emergency Physicians (tables of contents and abstracts).
- *Emergency Medical Abstract On Line* (http://www.ccme.org). Requires subscription.
- *Global Emergency Medicine Archives* (http://www.gema. library.ucsf.edu:8081). GEMA, an on-line medical journal from the Department of Emergency Medicine at Highland General Hospital in Oakland, California, and the Department of Emergency Medicine at the University of California at San Francisco.

Global Health Disaster Network.
- *Injury* (http://www.elsevier.com/locate/injury). Tables of contents.
- *Journal of the American Medical Association* (http://www.ama-assn.org/public/journals/jama/jamahome.htm).
- *Journal of Accident & Emergency Medicine* (http://www.bmjpg.com/data/aem.htm). Formerly *Archives of Emergency Medicine*. Tables of contents.
- *Journal of Emergency Medicine On-Line* (http://www.ccspublishing.com/j_er.htm).
- *Journal of Pediatric Medicine Online* (http://www.ccspublishing.com/j_ped.htm).
- *PEDIATRICS Electronic Pages* (http://www.pediatrics.org). *PEDIATRICS Electronic Pages* is the WWW extension of *Pediatrics,* the official journal of the American Academy of Pediatrics. This site contains exclusive new research articles covering advances in pediatric medicine. Users may also search back issues of *PEDIATRICS Electronic Pages,* review abstracts of articles published in the print version of *Pediatrics,* preview upcoming tables of contents for both the print version of *Pediatrics* and *PEDIATRICS Electronic Pages,* and review classified advertisements for professional opportunities.
- *Pediatric Emergency Care* (http://www.wwilkins.com/PEC).
- *Prehospital Immediate Care* (http://www.bmjpg.com/data/phic.htm). Tables of contents.
- *Prehospital Emergency Care* (http://www.hanleyandbelfus.com/journals/pec.html). *PEC,* the official journal of the National Association of EMS Physicians. Tables of contents.
- *The Completely Different Pediatric Emergency Medicine Journal* (http://pediatric-emergency.com/). Current research, reviews and critiques, data synthesis, and interesting cases.
- *The New England Journal of Medicine* (http://www.nejm.org/).
- *Weekly Web Review in Emergency Medicine* (http://www.wwrem.com/). Dedicated to the critical analysis of current clinical literature on topics relevant to the practice of emergency medicine; the reviews are updated each Friday.

Organizations

Many organizations have Web pages of varying complexity. Most

Web sites have information about future conferences, membership, links to related Web sites, and publications on-line.
- Ambulatory Pediatric Association Home Page (http://www. ambpeds.org/)
- **American Academy of Pediatrics (http://www.aap.org/)**
  - *Section on Emergency Medicine* (http://www.aap.org/ sections/semed.htm)
  - *Chapters*
    - ❖ California Chapter 1 of the AAP
    - ❖ California Chapter 2 of the AAP
    - ❖ District III of the AAP (http://www.aapdc.org/d3cr3_98.htm)
    - ❖ Georgia Chapter of the AAP (http://www.gaaap.org/gcp_ Home.htm)
    - ❖ Louisiana Chapter of the American Academy of Pediatrics (http://www.laaap.org/.)
    - ❖ Maryland Chapter of the AAP (http://www.med.jhu.edu/ mdaap.)
    - ❖ New Hampshire Pediatric Society (http://www.nhps.org/.)
    - ❖ New York Chapter 1 of the AAP (http://www.concentric.net/ ~ kidsmd/.)
    - ❖ Ohio Chapter of the AAP (http://www.ohioaap.org/)
    - ❖ Oregon Pediatric Society (http://www.ohsu.edu/som-Pediatrics/ops/ops.htm)
    - ❖ Pennsylvania Chapter of the AAP (http://www.voicenet. com/ ~ paaap/)
    - ❖ Uniformed Services East Chapter of the AAP (http://wpmc1. wpafb.af.mil/pages/peds/usce.html)
    - ❖ Vermont Chapter of the AAP (http://www.fahc.vtmednet. org/ ~ g125393/index.htm)
- American Association of Poison Control Centers (http://www. aapcc.org)
- American Board of Pediatrics (http://www.abp.org/.)
- American College of Physicians (http://www.acponline.org/)
- **American Heart Association** (http://www.amhrt.org/)
- American Medical Association (http://www.ama-assn.org/.)
- American Pediatric Society & Society for Pediatric Research (http://www.aps-spr.org/.)
- American Public Health Association (http://www.apha.org)
- Children's Defense Fund (http://www.childrensdefense.org/)

- **Children's Safety Network** (http://www.edc.org/HHD/csn/). The Children's Safety Network National Injury and Violence Prevention Resource Center is one of four children's safety resource centers funded by the Maternal and Child Health Bureau, US Department of Human and Health Services. This site offers injury-prevention publications on-line and by mail, as well as links to many injury-prevention resources on the WWW.
- **Emergency Medical Services for Children** (http://www.ems-c.org). A great site for information about EMS-C. Includes conference updates, contact information for EMS-C programs throughout the nation, grant information, and links to publications and Web sites.
- International Pediatric Association (http://www.urmc.rochester.edu/IPA/welcome.htm)
- International Society for Child and Adolescent Injury Prevention (http://www.weber.u.washington.edu/ ~ hiprc/iscaip.html)
- National Association of Pediatric Nurse Associates and Practitioners (http://www.napnap.org/)
- **National Center for Injury Prevention and Control** (http://www.cdc.gov/ncipc). This site offers access to information on research grants and funding opportunities, scientific data surveillance and injury statistics, publications, resources, and information about the National Center for Injury Prevention and Control.
- National Rural Health Services Research Database (http://www.muskie.usm.maine.edu/rhsrWelcome.htm). Database contains information on funded rural health services research projects under way.
- United States Public Health Service (http://www.phs.os.dhhs.gov/phs/phs.html)
  - Administration for Children and Families (http://www.acf.dhhs.gov/)
  - Agency for Health Care Policy and Research (http://www.ahcpr.gov)
  - Agency for Toxic Substances and Disease Registry (http://atsdr1.atsdr.cdc.gov:8080/atsdrhome.html)
  - Centers for Disease Control and Prevention (CDC) (http://www.cdc.gov)

- Food and Drug Administration (http://www.fda.gov/default. htm)
- Health Care Financing Administration (http://www.hcfa. gov/). Medicare and Medicaid.
- Health Resources and Services Administration (http:// www.hrsa.dhhs.gov/)
- Indian Health Service (http://www.tucson.ihs.gov/)
- National Institutes of Health (NIH) (http://www.nih.gov/)
- Substance Abuse and Mental Health Services Administration (http://www.samhsa.gov/)
- Society for Adolescent Medicine (http://cortex.uchc. edu/ ~ sam/)
- Society for Developmental and Behavioral Pediatrics (http://www. webcom.com/rusleepy/sdbp.html.)
- Society of Pediatric Nurses (http://www.pednurse.org/)

Research

The WWW is valuable for the EMS-C community engaged in research. The net offers a clearinghouse of information with many on-line databases. Investigators can access private and federal agencies, investigate past research and funding opportunities, and even apply for funding.

Databases

Many databases are available on the Internet. The ease of use among on-line databases varies widely. These sites accommodate either direct access to a database or requests for print information. Often, there is a contact person, and making use of that person's expertise is strongly suggested if you have any problems.

- *CDC Wonder* (http://wonder.cdc.gov). Data and document access from the CDC (mortality and morbidity).
- *DAWN's Estimates of Drug-Related Emergency-Department Episodes* (http://www.health.org/survey.htm). From the National Clearinghouse for Alcohol and Drug Information.
- *ER Watch* (http://www.erwatch.com). A searchable database of consumer product-related emergency-department cases derived from the US Consumer Product Safety Commission (CPSC), NEISS system. CPSC has not yet made its injury-surveillance data searchable on-line, but an entrepreneurial effort

by a health communications firm has begun to do so, although for now in a limited way (no weighting, no cross references, limited time periods). ER Watch is sponsored by Health Link Communications, a health and wellness communications firm.

- *Fatal Analysis Reporting System Database* (http://www.bts. gov/ntda/farsdb). From the US Department of Transportation. The Fatality Analysis Reporting System (FARS) contains data on all crashes in the United States (available by state) that occur on a public roadway and there is a fatality. Through this Web interface, FARS data are searchable and downloadable.
- *Health Statistics (University of Michigan)* (http://www.lib. umich.edu/libhome/Documents.center/sthealth.html).
- *Health, United States, 1996–1997, and Injury Chartbook* (http://www.cdc.gov/nchs/data/hus96_97.pdf). A 3.6-MB Adobe Acrobat file prepared by the National Center for Health Statistics, CDC, contains a comprehensive profile of injuries in the United States. 328 pp. (PHS) 96-1232. GPO stock number 017-022-01377-1.
- *Infant and Child Health Statistical Tables* (http://www.cdc.gov/ nchs/datawh/statab/pubd.htm). Data on breastfeeding, infant mortality, low birth weight, and prenatal care.
- *Injury Mortality Statistics from CDC* (http://www.cdc.gov/ ncipc/osp/mortdata.htm).
- *Injury Visits to US Emergency Departments, 1992, National Center for Health Statistics Advance Data Publication* (ftp://www. ftp.pitt.edu/users/h/w/hweiss/icrin/ad261.pdf). 214K Adobe Acrobat PDF file.
- *Inventory of Federal Data Systems in the United States for Injury Surveillance, Research, and Prevention Activities* (http://www.cdc. gov/ncipc/pub-res/federal.pdf). In Adobe Acrobat format. The document is more than 120 pages in length.
- *Leading Causes of Death* (http://www.cdc.gov/ncipc/osp/ 10lc92c.htm).
- *National Center for Health Statistics* (NCHS) (http://www. cdc.gov/ nchs/nchshome.htm). Excellent Web page containing news releases, publications, and information about the NCHS.
- *National Clearinghouse on Child Abuse and Neglect Information* (http://www.calib.com/nccanch/services/stats.htm). Key sta-

tistics from these studies are summarized in the National Child Abuse and Neglect Statistical Fact Sheet and In Fact.

- *The National EMS-C Data Analysis Resource Center* (NEDARC) (http://www-nedarc.med.utah.edu/nedarc). NEDARC is located at the University of Utah School of Medicine. Through a cooperative agreement with the Maternal and Child Health Bureau, NEDARC will provide technical assistance with the collection, maintenance, and analysis of high-quality data related to the care of children within the overall EMS system.
- *National Injury Mortality Statistics* (http://www.cdc.gov/ncipc/osp/usmort.htm).
- *The National Pediatric Trauma Registry* (http://www.nemc.org/rehab/nptrhome.htm). A multicenter, nationwide pediatric trauma registry established in 1985 to study the etiology of pediatric trauma and its consequences.
- *The Pediatric Database* (http://www.icondata.com/health/pedbase/index.htm). PEDBASE contains descriptions of more than 550 childhood disorders obtained from at least three sources, including the *Nelson Textbook of Pediatrics* (14th and 15th editions), the *Birth Defects Encyclopedia* (1990 and 1994 editions), and at least one other source (journal articles, review articles, textbooks).
- *State Injury Mortality* (http://www.wonder.cdc.gov/rchtml/Convert/data/injury.html).

Research Funding

Many Web sites offer information on research funding. The federal government has several well-developed sites such as the NIH Web site, which offers guidelines for funding applications, contact persons, and agency trends on project funding. Many privately supported sites also offer grant-writing tips and resources for applicants. Many grant application forms can be downloaded and, in the near future, on-line submissions will be commonplace.

- At-A-Glance Guide to Grants (http://www.sai.com/adjunct/nafg-grant.html).
- Government resources (http://www.os.dhhs.gov/progorg/grantsnet/otheruse/index.html).
- Federal Information Exchange (http://web.fie.com/ fedix/ index. html). Searchable index and automated alert for funding.

- Federal Register (http://www.access.gpo.gov/su_docs/aces/aces 140.html). The official source for federal grant announcements.
- FedWorld (http://www.fedworld.gov). A large site with search capabilities for many federal agencies.
- Foundation Center (http://www.fdncenter.org/).
- Government Printing Office (http://www.access.gpo.gov/su_docs/). The place to download grant applications and request or download government publications.
- Minority scholarships and fellowships (http://www.fie.com/molis/scholar.htm).
- National Academy of Sciences (http://www.nas.edu/).
- **The NIH** (http://www.nih.gov). A large Web site with valuable information. The following list includes some very useful pages at the NIH Web site.
  - NIH search engine (http://www.search.info.nih.gov). Searches the NIH Web site.
  - Grants Page/Office of Extramural Research (http://www.nih.gov/grants/oer.htm). Information on NIH extramural research and training programs including NIH funding opportunities (with application kits), grant policy, and access to the CRISP (Computer Retrieval of Information on Scientific Projects) database.
  - Award data (http://www.nih.gov/grants/award/award.htm). Contains data from NIH grants (1986–1995). Tables are arranged by Institute with success ratings/type of application, overall approval ratings, and much more.
  - CRISP (http://www-commons.cit.nih.gov/crisp/). Currently available on the Internet as a GOPHER-based system and CD-ROM, CRISP is a major biomedical database system containing information on research projects and programs supported by the Department of Health and Human Services.
  - NIH Health Information Index (http://www.nih.gov/news/96index/pubinae.htm). An alphabetical listing of topics and the institutions that have supported research ranging from acupuncture to zoonoses.
  - Alphabetical list of publications and databases (http://www.nih.gov/grants/documentindex.htm).
- National Science Foundation (http://www.nsf.gov/).
- NSF Career Planning Center (http://www.nas.edu/cpc/ index. html).

- Search for NSF grants (http://www.nsf.gov/verity/srchawd.htm).
- Preaward grant information (http://www.uth.tmc.edu/ut_general/research_acad_aff/ors/index.htm).
- The National Center for Education in Maternal and Child Health (http://www.ncemch.gerogetown.edu).
- US Department of Health and Human Services (http://www.os.dhhs.gov/).
- US federal, state, and local grant funding opportunities (http://www.statelocal.gov/funding.html).

Becoming a Presence on the Internet

Many people think that building a Web site is an enormous task requiring a large degree of technical skill. As the Internet has become easier to use, it has also become easier to place a Web site on the Web. Many Internet service providers offer free Web-site hosting, and many easy to use Web-site-creation programs exist. Web-site-creation programs reduce building a Web site to typing and formatting much like the typing and formatting of a normal document. Many private practices are putting Web sites on the Internet, as are hospitals and emergency departments. Advantages of having your own Web site include recruitment for a program, interaction with others in the community, and the ability to "place your message" on the Web to be accessed by the entire Internet community.

Summary

On-line services can help the primary-care physician find educational resources, gain clinical information, and network with other professionals.

Suggested Reading

Anthony D. *Health on the Internet.* Cambridge, MA: Blackwell Science; 1996

Coiera E. *Guide to Medical Informatics, the Internet, and Telemedicine.* New York, NY: Chapman and Hall; 1997

Gibbs SR, Sullivan-Fowler M, Rowe NW. *Mosby's Medical Safari: A Guide to Exploring the Internet and Discovering the Top Health Care Resources.* St Louis, MO: Mosby; 1996

Hutchinson D. *A Pocket Guide to the Medical Internet.* 2nd ed. Sacramento, CA: New Wind Publications; 1997

McKenzie BC. *Medicine and the Internet: Introducing Online Resources and Terminology.* 2nd ed. Oxford, UK, New York, NY: Oxford University Press; 1997

Pareras LG. *Medicine and the Internet.* Boston, MA: Little, Brown; 1996

Smith RP, Edwards MJA. *The Internet for Physicians.* 2nd ed. New York, NY: Springer Verlag; 1999

Stevenson T, Venditto G. Under construction. *Internet World.* 1997:8:73–85 (Review of Web-site authoring programs)

Part III

Hospital Preparation

The pediatrician works in many settings. One is the hospital. Not all hospitals are equal and not all have the same capacity to attend to the special needs of children. Organizing the hospital for EMS-C means 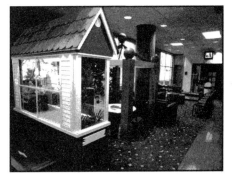 ensuring a child-friendly environment, the availability of equipment, and the use of child-specific protocols, which promote optimal care. This part of the book helps direct the pediatrician in achieving these goals.

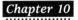

Chapter 10

The Community Hospital Emergency Department

Important Features of the Community Emergency Department

1. Should be staffed by qualified nurses and physicians.
2. Must be equipped and supplied for pediatric emergency care.
3. Must have pediatric-specific policies, procedures, and protocols.
4. Must have transfer agreements with pediatric receiving facilities.

Introduction

The public has an expectation that, if a hospital has an emergency department, it is prepared to manage all emergencies, including pediatric emergencies, 24 hours a day. Educate yourself and your patients that the ability of an institution in the community to respond appropriately to the needs of infants, children, and young adults may vary. The majority of pediatric emergency department visits are made by patients who are brought to the emergency department by a caretaker and not through the EMS system. The capability of a community emergency department to deliver pediatric emergency care depends on many factors. These factors include available equipment and supplies, training and experience of the staff, physical plant, availability of pediatric and surgical consultants, and formal links to higher levels of care. Facilities may be categorized by using a number of methods, some formal and governed by law or regulation, others voluntary and dependent on the commitment of the hospital. The definitions for facility categorization are given in Table 12.

Systems of care are often developed on the basis of facility categorization. Neonatal care is the oldest developed system of facilities categorization and has clearly been shown to influence outcome in certain types of high-risk neonates. Likewise, trauma systems have improved outcomes for injured adults and pediatric patients. Categorization of pediatric facilities, except for the de facto presence of a free-standing children's hospital, in the com-

Table 12.

Methods of Facility Categorization

Model	Definition
Categorization	Assessment of a facility based on its ability to manage certain categories of patients. Examples include burn centers, trauma centers, poison control centers, and level III neonatal intensive care centers.
Designation	The assignment of responsibility for care of certain categories of patients to specific institutions based on compliance with standards as well as on catchment area or other criteria.
Confirmation	An institution voluntarily agrees to adopt a set of standards as its own standard. It confirms that it has met a standard to care for a certain category of patient.

munity is in the early development stages. Los Angeles county's EMS system was the first to include specific pediatric destination policies for ambulances based on categorization of pediatric facilities. There are two levels of care: an Emergency Department Approved for Pediatrics (EDAP) and a Pediatric Critical Care Center (PCCC). Hospitals that are part of the Los Angeles county system have demonstrated a commitment to pediatric care by confirming that they meet a standard as defined by the county EMS agency, the Los Angeles Pediatric Society, and California Chapter 2 COPEM joint standard. Most of the acute-care hospitals in Los Angeles county are EDAPs, and there are nine PCCCs. The EDAP model can be used to best describe a community emergency department with pediatric commitment. The 1999 EDAP standards can be found in the Appendix at the end of this chapter. The basic philosophy of the EDAP is that an emergency department must have pediatric-appropriate equipment and supplies, be staffed by physicians and nurses skilled in pediatric emergency care, have pediatric-specific policies and procedures, and be linked by formalized transfer agreements to PCCCs (see

Chapter 12). Transportation guidelines help base-hospital personnel and out-of-hospital physicians triage pediatric patients on the basis of criteria for trauma or medical illness.

Other states, regions, and municipalities are beginning to examine the pediatric capabilities of the community hospitals. A consensus group sponsored by the Health Resources and Services Administration (HRSA), Maternal and Child Health Bureau, has developed a list of minimum equipment and supplies for emergency departments (see Table 13). Comparing the equipment and supplies available in your community emergency department with the list is a good beginning in examining your emergency department's preparedness for pediatric emergency care.

Table 13.

Essential and Desirable Emergency Department Equipment and Supplies

Monitoring

Cardiorespiratory monitor with strip recorder
Defibrillator (0–400 joules capability) with pediatric and adult paddles (4.5 cm and 8 cm)
Pediatric and adult monitor electrodes
Pulse oximeter with sensor sizes from newborn through adult
Thermometer/rectal probe[1]
Sphygmomanometer
Doppler blood pressure device
Blood pressure cuffs (neonatal, infant, child, adult, and thigh sizes)
Method to monitor endotracheal tube and placement [2]

Vascular Access

Butterfly needles (sizes 19–25 gauge)
Catheter-over-needle devices (sizes 14–24 gauge)
Infusion device[3]
Tubing for infusion device
Intraosseous needles (sizes 16 and 18 gauge)[4]
Arm boards (infant, child, and adult sizes)
IV fluid/blood warmer[5]
Umbilical vein catheters (sizes 3.5 and 5F)[6]

continued

Seldinger technique vascular access kit (with pediatric sizes 3, 4, and 5F catheters)

Airway Management

Clear oxygen masks (preterm, infant, child, and adult sizes)
Nonrebreathing masks (infant, child, and adult sizes)
Oral airways (sizes 00–5)
Nasopharyngeal airways (12–30F)
Bag-valve-mask resuscitator, self-inflating (450- and 1000-ml sizes)
Nasal cannulae (infant, child, and adult sizes)
Endotracheal tubes, uncuffed (sizes 2.5–5.5) and cuffed (sizes 5.5–9)
Stylets (pediatric and adult sizes)
Laryngoscope handle (pediatric and adult)
Laryngoscope blades, curved (sizes 2 and 3) and straight (sizes 0–3)
Magill forceps (pediatric and adult)
Nasogastric tubes (sizes 6–14F)
Suction catheters, flexible: sizes 5–16F and Yankauer suction tip
Chest tubes (sizes 8–40F)
Tracheostomy tubes (sizes 00–6)[7]

Resuscitation Medications

Medication chart, tape, or other system to ensure ready access to information on proper per kilogram doses for resuscitation drugs and equipment sizes[8]

Miscellaneous

Infant and standard scales
Infant formula and oral rehydrating solutions
Heating source[9]
Towel rolls/blanket rolls or equivalent
Pediatric restraining devices
Resuscitation board
Sterile linen[10]

Specialized Pediatric Trays

Tube thoracotomy with water seal drainage capability
Lumbar puncture (spinal needle sizes 20, 22, and 25 gauge)
Urinary catheterization with pediatric Foley catheters (sizes 5–16F)

continued

Obstetrical pack
Newborn kit
  umbilical vessel cannulation supplies
  meconium aspirator
Venous cutdown
Surgical airway kit[11]

Fracture Management

Cervical immobilization equipment (sizes child–adult)[12]
Extremity splints
Femur splints (child and adult sizes)

Desirable Equipment and Supplies

Medical photography capability

....

[1] Suitable for hypothermic and hyperthermic measurements with temperature capability from 25° to 44°C

[2] May be satisfied by a disposable $ETCO_2$ detector, bulb or feeding tube methods for endotracheal tube placement.

[3] To regulate rate and volume.

[4] May be satisfied by standard bone marrow aspiration needles, 13 or 15 gauge.

[5] Available within the hospital.

[6] Available within the hospital.

[7] Ensure availability of pediatric sizes within the hospital.

[8] System for estimating medication doses and supplies may use the length-based method with color codes or other predetermined weight (kg/dose) method.

[9] May be met by infrared lamps or overhead warmer.

[10] Available within hospital for burn care.

[11] May include any of the following items: tracheostomy tray, cricothyrotomy tray, ETJV (needle jet).

[12] Many types of cervical immobilization devices are available. They include wedges and collars. The type of device chosen will depend on local preference and policies and procedures. Whatever device is chosen should be stocked in sizes to fit infants, children, adolescents, and adults. The use of sandbags to meet this requirement is discouraged because they may cause injury if the patient has to be turned.

The equipment and supply guidelines presented in Table 13 are minimal. An emergency department may choose to modify this list to meet the acuity level of the patient population. Emergency departments that see a high volume of ill and injured pediatric patients may need additional items not on this list. In the purchase of equipment and supplies, consideration should be given to the growing problem of latex sensitization of both patients and healthcare workers. The use of hypoallergenic materials for both routine and special pediatric procedures is encouraged.

Staffing

Not all community emergency departments are staffed by physicians and nurses who have experience and training in pediatric emergency care. If the physician staff is residency trained in emergency medicine or pediatrics, they will have had preparation in resuscitation and the management of most pediatric emergencies. Physicians who are not prepared in these specialties should, at a minimum, be trained in Pediatric Advanced Life Support (PALS) or Advanced Pediatric Life Support (APLS) or both.

Many emergency department nurses are not trained in pediatric emergency care. Surveys clearly demonstrate that they are particularly uncomfortable in caring for infants and young children. At least one nurse on duty each shift should be PALS prepared. Encourage all the nursing staff to take the self-learning course or the Emergency Nursing Pediatric Course (ENPC) offered by the Emergency Nurses Association (ENA; see Chapter 2).

Every emergency department should have a call panel that includes pediatricians. If there is no pediatrician in the community, there should be a policy and procedure in place to obtain consultation from the regional pediatric receiving center. Pediatricians should participate with emergency physicians in the development of practice management guidelines, policies, and procedures used for pediatric care.

Policies, Procedures, and Protocols

Assist your local emergency department in establishing pediatric policies, procedures, and protocols that are family centered and promote high-quality emergency care. They might cover the following topics:
- Triage and initial evaluation
- Patient safety
- Suspected child abuse and neglect
- Family violence
- Consent for treatment
- Sedation and analgesia
- Transfer for higher level of care to a pediatric referral center

- Telephone consultation with pediatric specialists
- Do-not-resuscitate (DNR)
- Death of a child
- Sudden infant death syndrome (SIDS) and apparent life-threatening event (ALFE)
- Aeromedical transport to include landing procedures
- Daily verification of proper location and functioning of equipment and supplies
- Immunizations
- Parental presence during procedures
- Ground transport procedures and physicians

The community emergency department should have written interfacility transfer agreements with regional trauma, pediatric referral, burn, and other specialized centers (see Chapter 12).

Quality Improvement

Pediatric quality improvement should be part of the emergency department quality-improvement plan and activities. Local pediatricians may wish to participate in the organization and management of the quality-improvement activities. Suggested topics for quality-improvement review include:

- Deaths
- Cardiac and respiratory arrest
- Suspected child abuse and neglect
- Transfers to or from another facility or both
- Admissions to the operating room or intensive care unit
- Selected return visits to the emergency department within 48 hours of the original visit
- Pediatric EMS transports

Support Services

Support services available in community hospitals must include pediatric capabilities. These services include respiratory care, radiology, and microtechnique laboratory services.

Outpatient Extended-Treatment Sites

Some emergency departments have developed extended-treatment sites or observation units where children who require extended therapy can be observed and monitored without being hospitalized. Some of these units are in the emergency department or adjacent to it, whereas others are on the same floor but separate from the in-patient unit. They are staffed by dedicated nursing and physician staff and manage a variety of illnesses, including:

- Acute asthma
- Diarrhea, vomiting, and dehydration
- Mild diabetic ketoacidosis
- Acute abdominal pain
- Parenteral antibiotic administration

One study found that an estimated 70% of the admissions for acute asthma could have been managed in an extended-treatment site in the course of two nursing shifts (16 hours). These units are less expensive than inpatient units and are an alternative to traditional inpatient care.

Summary

Not all emergency departments are prepared to offer high-quality pediatric emergency care. The role of the pediatrician in ensuring that children have high-quality emergency care begins with an examination of the capabilities of the community hospital emergency department. Aspects to be examined include:

- Equipment
- Staffing
- Policies, procedures, and protocols for pediatric emergency care
- Participation in quality improvement
- Support services that include pediatric capabilities
- A system of transporting patients who require a higher level of pediatric care to appropriate facilities

Suggested Reading

American Academy of Pediatrics, Committee on Pediatric Emergency Medicine. Guidelines for pediatric emergency care facilities. *Pediatrics.* 1995;96:526–537

Dieckmann RA, ed. *Pediatric Emergency Care Systems: Planning and Management.* Baltimore, MD: Williams & Wilkins; 1992

Durch JS, Lohr KN, eds. *Emergency Medical Services for Children: Institute of Medicine Report.* Washington, DC: National Academy Press; 1993

Emergency Medical Services Authority, State of California. *Emergency Medical Services for Children: Final Report.* Sacramento, CA: Emergency Medical Services Authority; 1994

Henderson DP. The Los Angeles pediatric emergency care system. *J Emerg Nurs.* 1988;14:96–100

McConnochie KM, Russo MJ, McBride JT, Szilagyi PG, Brooks AM, Roghmann KJ. How commonly are children hospitalized for asthma eligible for care in alternative settings? *Arch Pediatr Adolesc Med.* 1999;153:49–55

Seidel JS, Henderson DP, eds. *Emergency Medical Services for Children: A Report to the Nation.* Washington, DC: National Center for Education in Maternal and Child Health; 1991

Seidel JS, Henderson DP, Lewis JB. Emergency medical services and the pediatric patient III: resources of ambulatory care centers. *Pediatrics.* 1991;88:230–235

Seidel J, Tittle S, Hodge D 3rd, et al. Guidelines for pediatric equipment and supplies for emergency departments. *Ann Emerg Med.* 1998;31:54–57, *Pediatr Emerg Care.* 1998;14:62–64, *J Emerg Nurs.* 1998;24:45–48

Wiley JF II, Friday JH, Nowakowski T, Pittsinger-Kazimer L, Platt K, Scribano PV. Observation units: the role of an outpatient extended treatment site in pediatric care. *Pediatr Emerg Care.* 1998;14:444–447

Appendix

1999 LOS ANGELES COUNTY DEPARTMENT OF HEALTH SERVICES EMERGENCY MEDICAL SERVICES AGENCY EDAP STANDARDS

INTRODUCTION:

These standards were developed as a concerted effort by the Committee on Pediatric Emergency Medicine which is made up of representatives from the following organizations: Los Angeles Pediatric Society, Pediatric Liaison Nurses of Los Angeles County, California Chapter of the American College of Emergency Physicians, National EMSC Resource Alliance, California Chapter 2 of the American Academy of Pediatrics, Emergency Nurses Association, American College of Surgeons, and Los Angeles County Department of Health Services Emergency Medical Services Agency.

These standards have been approved by The Health Care Association of Southern California and meet or exceed Emergency Medical Services for Children (EMSC) administration, personnel, and policy guidelines for the care of pediatric patients in the emergency department set forth by the California Emergency Medical Services Authority in 1995.

DEFINITIONS:

Emergency Department Approved for Pediatrics (EDAP): A licensed basic emergency department that is approved by the County of Los Angeles to receive pediatric patients from the 9-1-1 system. These emergency departments provide care to pediatric patients by meeting specific requirements for professional staff, quality improvement, education, support services, equipment, supplies, medications, and established policies, procedures, and protocols.

Board prepared/eligible: Successful completion of a Board approved emergency medicine or pediatric residency training program.

Promptly available: Being in the emergency department within a period of time that is medically prudent and appropriate to the patient's clinical condition; and further, that the interval between the arrival of the patient to the emergency department and the arrival of the respondent should not have a measurably harmful effect on the course of patient management or outcome.

Qualified specialist: A physician licensed in the State of California who has: 1) taken special postgraduate medical training, or has met other specified requirements; and 2) has become board certified within six years of qualification for board certification in the corresponding speciality for those specialities that have board certification and are recognized by the American Board of Medical Specialities.

Senior resident: A physician licensed in the State of California who has completed at least two years of the residency under consideration and has the capability of initiating treatment when the clinical situation demands, and who is in training as a member of the residency program at the designated hospital.

PALS: American Heart Association Pediatric Advanced Life Support Course.

APLS: American Academy of Pediatrics-American College of Emergency Physicians Advanced Pediatric Life Support Course

ENPC: Emergency Nurses Association-Emergency Nursing Pediatric Course

I. ADMINISTRATION/COORDINATION
    A. EDAP Medical Director
        1. Qualifications:
            a. Qualified specialist in Emergency Medicine or Pediatrics
            b. Current PALS or APLS physician
        2. Responsibilities:
            a. Oversight of EDAP quality improvement (QI) program
            b. Member of hospital emergency department committee and pediatric committee
            c. Liaison with pediatric critical care centers (PCCC), trauma centers, base hospitals, community hospitals, prehospital care physicians, and the EMS Agency
            d. Identify needs and facilitate pediatric education for emergency department physicians

e. Review, approve, and assist in development of all pediatric policies and procedures

B. Designated Pediatric Consultant

1. Qualifications: Board certified in pediatrics or having completed the written exam and actively pursuing Board certification in pediatrics.

2. Responsibilities:

   a. Member of hospital emergency department committee and pediatric committee

   b. Participation with EDAP staff in developing and monitoring pediatric QI program, protocols, and policies and procedures

   c. Consult with EDAP Medical Director and Pediatric Liaison Nurse as needed

NOTE: Pediatric Consultant may also be EDAP Medical Director

C. Pediatric Liaison Nurse (PdLN)

1. Qualifications:

   a. At least two years experience in pediatrics or in an emergency department that sees pediatric patients, within the previous five years

   b. Experience with QI programs is recommended

   c. Current PALS or APLS physician or ENPC course

   d. Completion of a two day pediatric emergency nursing course*

   e. Completion of eight hours of Board of Registered Nursing (BRN) approved continuing education units (CEU) in pediatric topics every two years

*NOTE: A two day pediatric emergency nursing course should include a broad spectrum of topics including: resuscitation, trauma, medical conditions, near drowning, respiratory distress, ingestion, child abuse and neglect, fever, seizures, and neonatal emergencies.

2. Responsibilities:

   a. Attend monthly meetings of The Pediatric Liaison Nurses of Los Angeles County

   b. Participate in development and maintenance of pediatric QI program

   c. Liaison with PCCC's, trauma centers, base hospitals, community hospitals, prehospital care physicians, and the EMS Agency

d. Member of selected hospital based emergency department and/or pediatric committees

e. Notify the EMS Agency in writing of any change in status of the EDAP Medical Director, Pediatric Consultant, and Pediatric Liaison Nurse

II. **PERSONNEL**

A. Physicians-Qualifications/Education

1. Twenty four hour emergency department coverage shall be provided or directly supervised by physicians functioning as emergency physicians or pediatricians experienced in emergency care on a full time basis. (96 hours or more per month in an emergency department) This includes senior residents practicing at their respective hospitals only.

2. At least 75% of the emergency department coverage shall be provided by physicians Board certified or eligible in emergency medicine or pediatrics.

3. Those emergency department physicians who are not board certified or eligible shall be a current PALS or APLS physician.

B. Nurses-Qualifications/Education

1. At least 75% of the total RN staff and at least one RN per shift in the emergency department shall be a current PALS or APLS physician.

2. At least one RN per shift shall have completed a two day pediatric emergency nursing course (within the last 4 years).

NOTE: It is highly recommended that all nurses regularly assigned to the emergency department meet the above requirements.

3. All nurses assigned to the emergency department shall attend at a minimum, eight hours of pediatric BRN approved education every two years.

C. Pediatric physicians/Speciality services

1. Establishment of a pediatric on call panel that allows for telephone consultation and a promptly available pediatrician to the emergency department twenty

four hours per day. This pediatrician shall be Board certified or eligible.

2. A plan shall exist whereby other pediatric specialists may be consulted and available in at least the following specialities: surgery, orthopedics, anesthesia and neurosurgery. This requirement may be met by a written agreement with a PCCC.

3. A plan shall exist whereby a second emergency physician or pediatrician will be available within thirty minutes to serve as back-up for the emergency department in critical situations.

III. POLICIES, PROCEDURES, AND PROTOCOLS
A. Establish procedures, and protocols for pediatric emergency patients to include but not limited to:
1. Triage and initial evaluation
2. Patient safety
3. Suspected child abuse and neglect
4. Transfers
5. Consents
6. Conscious sedation
7. Do-not-resuscitate (DNR)
8. Death to include SIDS and the care of the grieving family
9. Aeromedical transport to include landing procedure
10. Daily verification of proper location and functioning of equipment and supplies
11. Immunizations
B. Establish a written interfacility consult and transfer agreement with a PCCC to facilitate transfers of critically ill and injured pediatric patients and twenty four hour telephone consultation.
C. Establish a written interfacility consult and transfer agreement with a California Children Services (CCS) approved Level II or Level III Neonatal Intensive Care Unit (NICU).

IV. QUALITY IMPROVEMENT (QI)
A. A pediatric QI program shall be developed and monitored by the EDAP Medical Director and Pediatric Liai-

son Nurse with input from the Designated Pediatric Consultant as needed.

B. The program should include an interface with prehospital care, emergency department, trauma, pediatric critical care, pediatric in-patient, and hospital wide QI activities.

C. A mechanism shall be established to easily identify pediatric (14 years & under) visits to the emergency department.

D. The pediatric QI program should include identification of the indicators, methods to collect data, results and conclusions, recognition of improvement, action(s) taken, assessment of effectiveness of above actions and communication process for participants.

E. The pediatric QI program should include review of the following pediatric patients seen in the emergency department:
   1. Deaths
   2. Cardiopulmonary and or respiratory arrests, including all pediatric intubations
   3. Suspected child abuse or neglect
   4. Transfers to and/or from another facility
   5. Admissions from the emergency department to an adult ward or ICU
   6. Selected return visits to the emergency department
   7. Pediatric transports within the 9-1-1 system

F. A mechanism to document and monitor pediatric education of EDAP staff will be established.

V. SUPPORT SERVICES

A. Respiratory Therapy
   1. At least one respiratory therapist shall be in house twenty four hours per day.
   2. Current PALS or APLS physician.

B. Radiology
   1. Radiologist on call and promptly available twenty four hour per day.
   2. Radiology technician in house twenty four hours per day with a second technician on call and promptly available.

3. CT scan technician on call and promptly available.
C. Laboratory
  1. Technician in house twenty four hours per day and a second technician on call and promptly available.
  2. Clinical Laboratory capabilities in house:
    a. Chemistry
    b. Hematology
    c. Blood bank
    d. Arterial blood gas
    f. Microbiology
    g. Toxicology
    h. Drug levels
    NOTE: Toxicology and drug levels may be done outside if routine tests are available within two hours.

VI. EQUIPMENT, SUPPLIES, AND MEDICATIONS

Pediatric equipment, supplies, and medications shall be easily accessible, labeled, and logically organized. EDAP staff shall be appropriately educated as to the locations of all items. Each EDAP shall have a method of daily verification of proper location and function of equipment and supplies. It is highly recommended that each EDAP have a mobile pediatric crash cart.

The following are requirements for equipment, supplies, and medications for an EDAP:

GENERAL EQUIPMENT
  Foley catheters (8–22 fr.)
  IV blood/fluid warmer
  Length and weight tape for determining pediatric resuscitation drug dosages
  Meconium Aspirator
  OB Kit
  Posted or readily available pediatric drug dosage reference material calculated on a dose per kilogram basis.
  Restraint device
  Scale
  Warming device

MONITORING EQUIPMENT
  Blood pressure cuffs (infant, child, adult, and thigh)

Doppler

ECG monitor/defibrillator (0–400 joules) with pediatric and adult paddles

End tidal CO_2 monitor or detector (adult and pediatric sizes)

Hypothermia thermometer

Pulse oximeter

RESPIRATORY EQUIPMENT

Bag-valve-mask device, self inflating (pediatric size: 450–900 ml and adult size: 1000–2000 ml)

Bag-valve masks, clear (neonate, infant, child, and adult sizes)

Endotracheal tubes (uncuffed: 2.5–5.5 and cuffed: 6.0–9.0)

Laryngoscope (curved and straight: 0–3)

Lubricant (water soluble)

Magill forceps (pediatric and adult)

Nasal cannulae (infant, child, and adult)

Nasopharyngeal airways (infant, child, adult)

Nasogastric tubes (including 5 and 8 fr feeding tubes)

Oral airways (sizes 0–5)

Oxygen masks, clear (standard and non-rebreathing) for infant, child, and adult

Stylets for endotracheal tubes

Suction catheters (sizes 6–12 fr)

Tracheostomy tubes (sizes 0–6)

Yankauer suction tips

VASCULAR ACCESS EQUIPMENT

Arm boards (infant, child, adult)

Butterfly needles (19–25 ga)

Central venous catheters (sizes 6–12 fr)

Infusion devices to regulate rate and volume

Intraosseous needles

IV administration sets with calibrated chambers

IV catheters (14–24 ga)

IV solutions (D5.2NS, D5.45NS, D5NS, D10W, and NS)

Needles (18–27 ga)

Stopcocks (3 way)

Syringes (TB and 1–60 cc)

T-connectors

Umbilical vein catheters (may substitute 5 fr feeding tube)

FRACTURE MANAGEMENT DEVICES
    Cervical spine immobilization devices
    Pediatric femur splint
    Spine board (long and short)
SPECIALIZED TRAYS
    Cricothyrotomy tray
    Pediatric lumbar puncture tray
    Pediatric thoracotomy tray
    Pediatric tracheostomy tray
    Peritoneal lavage tray
    Thoracostomy and chest tube tray (sizes 16–28 fr)
    Venous cutdown tray
RESUSCITATION MEDICATIONS
    Atropine
    Adenosine
    Bretylium
    Calcium chloride
    Dextrose (25% and 50%)
    Dopamine
    Dobutamine
    Epinephrine (1:1000 and 1:10,000)
    Flumazenol
    Lidocaine
    Naloxone
    Racemic epinephrine for inhalation
    Sodium Bicarbonate (8.4% and 4.2%)

NOTE: It is suggested that these drugs be immediately available in the resuscitation room and not locked in a computerized system.

Making the Environment Child Friendly

Tips for Making a Child-Friendly Environment

1. Separate children from adult patients and frightening sights and sounds.
2. Make décor bright, colorful, and age neutral.
3. Ensure a safe environment.
4. Provide distraction and entertainment.
5. Consider needs of adolescents.

Introduction

An emergency department treating children must address the needs and expectations of three constituencies: children, adolescents, and parents. Children are reassured by evidence that the emergency department is an environment capable of seeing the world through their eyes. Adolescents, on the other hand, desire an emergency department that understands that they are no longer children. Parents share the expectations of their children and adolescents, but they also demand professionalism. An environment that "works" for the child (murals of cartoon characters) will not necessarily satisfy adolescents or parents. This chapter considers the needs of these three groups and methods for addressing these needs within one facility.

Protection From Frightening Sights and Sounds

The child and adolescent must be separated at all times from the frightening sights and sounds that are part and parcel of a general emergency department. Such separation can be best accomplished with a facility that is completely separate from the emergency department treating adult patients: separate entrance, separate waiting area, and separate traffic pattern. However, even within an entirely separate area, additional consideration must be given to sheltering the child from unpleasant experiences. There should be a separate ambulance entrance. The traffic pattern from that ambulance entrance to the trauma and resuscitation room should not intersect the paths or rooms of other children. Upset family members should be secluded in a "quiet room" for both their own comfort and for the protection of other children and families in the emergency department. Finally, a soundproofed procedure room is an important part of any emergency department treating children. Although most procedures should be accomplished with minimal pain and, therefore, with minimal crying, the occasional upset or agitated child must be managed in a fashion that does not upset other children in the emergency department.

A design that works particularly well is the double-entrance examining room. One entrance leads to the nursing station—used by medical personnel. The other door leads directly to a waiting area. This design has the following advantages: (1) it minimizes the exposure of a given child to the events taking place in other examining rooms, (2) it maximizes staff privacy, and (3) it affords the extended family a means of remaining together while not overpopulating the examining room. This design, however, also has the following disadvantages: (1) it requires more square footage, (2) it is less secure, and (3) an upset or crying child can be easily heard in the waiting area.

Decor and Furniture

Bright colors appeal to children. They also relate well to basic shapes such as triangles, squares, and circles. Tastefully combining bright colors with basic shapes can create a decor that is satisfying for all age groups. Children's art that is professionally framed is another example of decor with universal appeal. Parents gaze at the pictures for an eternity searching for hidden meaning. Children simply look and smile. A final example of wall decor that is satisfying to all ages consists of convex and concave mirrors.

Furniture should have no sharp edges or corners, be colorful, and be easily cleaned. Some child-sized furniture is desirable as further demonstration to the child that he or she is in a child-friendly environment. Furniture should be arranged in small clusters to accommodate the desire of most families for privacy. In particular, parents are understandably often reluctant to have their children play with other children in an emergency department because of the risk of exposure to contagious disease. For this reason, play areas designed to be used by several children at one time are discouraged.

Safety

Just as we encourage parents to childproof their homes, so must we ensure that the emergency department that treats children is childproof. Carpeting is desirable in the waiting areas not only to reduce noise levels, but also to reduce the risk of injury from falls. Electrical sockets should be protected with self-closing covers. Wires in examining rooms should be out of reach. Of particular concern is making sure that small objects that could be aspirated are kept away from searching hands. Ear speculums, for example, should be stored in drawers or mounted high and away from the examining table. If toys are provided (the concern again is contagious disease), they should all pass safety standards for the youngest age groups.

The sharp container must be childproof and clearly out of reach. Similarly, all waste containers should be covered and tall. Cribs in ample supply are critical. Because the ratio of infants to older children varies from day to day, cribs that allow all four sides to be lowered are useful. The use of such cribs enables the examining room to accommodate a child in a fashion that does not suggest to the child that he or she is being treated like an infant.

A common piece of furniture in most examining rooms is a rolling stool. It is particularly useful in pediatrics for examining a child on a parent's lap. The stool allows the examiner to move easily around the child and adjust easily to the height of the child. The problem is that the stool poses a safety risk for the child. One solution is a strict policy that requires removal of the stool from the examining room when not in use and the room is occupied by a young child. It can be temporarily placed just outside the door.

Distraction and Entertainment

Waiting to be seen is never easy. Waiting for a long period of time with one or more small children can be unbearable without adequate means to distract and entertain the children. A television set with videocassette recorder (VCR) capabilities in every room is surprisingly inexpensive and pays remarkably high dividends, particularly when there is an ample supply of tapes that appeal to all age groups (including parents). The VCR can be an excellent tool for patient education. Tapes on asthma home care, wound care, and oral rehydration therapy are particularly useful.

Materials that encourage solo activity are highly desirable, both because much of the waiting is in individual examining rooms and because, again, individual activity in the waiting areas can reduce the spread of contagious disease. Coloring books, picture books, and reading books for various ages are useful but will need to be replenished frequently. A large variety is necessary. Parents become distressed when they have to read *The Cat in the Hat* 30 times to their child! Etch-a-Sketch and hand-held electronic games are ideal means of entertaining children beyond the toddler range. However, they are difficult to track and retrieve.

Distraction and entertainment is not only good public relations, but also good pediatric medicine. General appearance, the fifth vital sign of pediatrics, is more accurately assessed when the child's environment is normalized. Lacerations are more easily sewn without restraint and heavy sedation if a familiar character is there for the child. Stethoscopes go unnoticed when the examination takes place on the lap of a parent who is reading about Goofy's picnic.

Conveniences for Parents

Parents need to communicate with the outside world, feed their children, change their children's diapers, rock their infants to sleep in a warm blanket, and (most important and often forgotten) be able to leave their child briefly (use the bathroom, get the car seat from the car, etc.). Communication needs are met by having a telephone in *every* examining room and linked to an operator who can assist with long-distance calls. The solution to feeding the infant and young child is not waiting an hour for a special meal or formula to be delivered from the hospital kitchen. Try telling a hungry infant or toddler that dinner will be served in an hour! The emergency department needs to stock ample supplies and varieties of infant formulas, juices, crackers, and so forth. And a coffee machine for the parent will pay great dividends when an impatient parent is perceiving the world at large and your emergency department as uncaring.

Rockers in every room can be cumbersome. However, parents of infants are grateful for a few rocking chairs that can be easily moved from room to room. Finally, cribs and personnel who readily offer to watch infants and small children during a parent's absence are critical to enabling the parent to leave the child briefly.

Professionalism

A copy of *The Cat in the Hat*, "Barney" on the VCR, crayons, and crackers all reassure the child. However, if the crayons are thrown about, the book is missing its cover, and the doctor is dressed to go to the beach (ostensibly so as not to frighten the child by wearing a uniform), the parent is not reassured that the emergency department provides high-quality medical care. In other words, creating a child-friendly environment inherently tends to compromise the professional atmosphere that is also expected by parents. Extra efforts must be made to guarantee neatness, cleanliness, and professional, albeit child-friendly, behavior on the part of the emergency department staff. Efforts to prevent the spread of contagious disease through strict hand-washing and wiping down toys brought to the room are examples of professional behavior that do not go unnoticed by parents.

Staff should be well versed in dealing with various age groups. Bright colors, toys, and rocking chairs are all for naught if the triage nurse stands forebodingly over a 3-year-old child with a small facial laceration, insisting that his clothes be removed so that his blood pressure can be taken.

Laboratory coats are controversial. Admittedly, the laboratory coat frightens a small number of children. However, studies suggest that the number is smaller than generally believed. If the physicians and nurses choose to forgo white laboratory coats and uniforms, then their dress should be otherwise impeccable. Parents may tolerate their private pediatrician in a sport shirt and jeans because they have known him for years and look past the clothes into his true self. However, parents and children are meeting emergency department personnel for the first time and are searching for clues about the expertise and professionalism of the people who are about to offer care. Studies have clearly demonstrated that parents have more confidence in caregivers who are well dressed. Another perspective on the laboratory coat is the signal that it sends to both parents and children. It defines a role. It states that the wearer is committed to that role. And it helps children to understand why this person is touching him or her in ways that others have not been allowed.

Although most emergency department physicians and nurses wear scrub tops and pants, studies have shown that both parents and children prefer physicians who are dressed in shirts, ties, and white coats.

Adolescents

Adolescents desire privacy, an understanding that they are not children, and a selection of entertainment and distractions that do not begin with Mickey Mouse and end with Barney. Sectioning the waiting area into small units where an adolescent with or without his or her family can be away from small children is desirable. If one or two of these areas also has computers loaded with both games and medical education "brain teasers," all the better. The medical history and examination of the adolescent should always take place in a private examining room, not in an area with multiple bays separated by curtains. The adolescent girl presenting herself to triage as merely having a sore throat may also be seeking treatment for a vaginal discharge. Finally, adolescents may prefer a medical evaluation without an accompanying parent present. This preference should be offered routinely to older adolescents. The examiner should always be chaperoned by a staff member.

Policies and Procedures

Just as adolescents often wish to be examined without a parent present, children will almost always tolerate medical evaluation and procedures better in the presence of a parent. Any child-friendly environment will not only have the latter as policy but will also encourage parents to remain with their children during procedures. In fact, many procedures, ranging, for example, from visualization of the middle ear to the repair of selected lacerations, are best performed in a parent's arms or lap. To accomplish this goal, written policy is not sufficient. Emergency department personnel must be comfortable with parents being present during procedures. Many emergency departments permit parental presence during trauma resuscitation and cardiopulmonary resuscitation (CPR; see Chapter 13).

All of the policies and procedures that promote a child-friendly environment are too numerous to list and present in detail. However, the following partial list of matters that must be addressed illustrates the breadth and detail of a policy and procedure manual that strives to foster a child-friendly environment: dealing with the frightened child in triage (vital signs, gowning, ID bracelet), methods of administering medications to the unwilling infant or toddler, pain control and sedation, and the rights of minor children.

Summary

Creating a child-friendly environment is not simply painting cartoon characters on the walls. In fact, that would be a blatant mistake! And, even if appropriate decor, furniture, and distractions are chosen, the emergency department or office will fail in its mission to the child if it is not populated with personnel who are inherently friendly to children and governed by policies and procedures that define and provide quality-assurance measures of child-friendly behavior and actions.

Most community hospitals do not have separate pediatric emergency departments. However, steps can be taken to provide a separate waiting area for children, as well as appropriate space for their clinical care. Suggestions made in this chapter are applicable to all general emergency departments.

Suggested Reading

Bauchner H, Vinci R, Bak S, Pearson C, Corwin MJ. Parents and procedures: a randomized controlled trial. *Pediatrics.* 1996;98:861–867

Gonzalez Del Rey JA, Paul RI. Preferences of parents for pediatric emergency physicians' attire. *Pediatr Emerg Care.* 1995;11:361–364

Marino RV, Rosenfeld W, Narula P, Karakurum M. Impact of pediatricians' attire on children and parents. *J Dev Behav Pediatr.* 1991;12:98–101

Matsui D, Cho M, Rieder MJ. Physicians' attire as perceived by young children and their parents: the myth of the white coat syndrome. *Pediatr Emerg Care.* 1998;14:198–201

Sacchetti A, Lichenstein R, Carraccio CA, Harris RH. Family member presence during pediatric emergency department procedures. *Pediatr Emerg Care.* 1996;12:268–271

The Pediatric Critical Care Center

Important Facts About Pediatric Critical Care Centers

1. There are different levels of receiving centers.

2. Receiving centers provide consultation, education, communication, and coordination of care.

3. Written transfer agreements should be in place.

Introduction

The pediatric critical care center (PCCC) plays an important role in providing specialized personnel, facilities, and services for children. In the past decade, there have been a number of important changes in the care of critically ill and injured children. These changes have taken place on many fronts and are the result of the efforts of many organizations and agencies. Pediatric emergency and critical care training programs and training programs leading to board certification in the subspecialties of critical care and pediatric emergency medicine have produced highly qualified physicians with expertise in the stabilization and management of critically ill and injured children. Pediatric and family medicine residency training programs provide exposure to these children for physicians in training in both the emergency department and the pediatric intensive care unit (PICU). Such formal rotations were not widely available 20 years ago. Specialized training programs have also been developed for other members of the healthcare team, such as nurses and respiratory therapists.

Historically, pediatricians and community hospitals have referred patients to centers that have been able to provide specialized pediatric care and expertise (such as neonatology, cardiology, and hematology/oncology). Through time, these same receiving centers have evolved to include sophisticated emergency departments approved for pediatrics (EDAPs), PCCCs, and PICUs that have the capability of caring for the critically ill and injured child.

Professional organizations such as the American Academy of

Pediatrics (AAP) and the Society for Critical Care Medicine (SCCM) have worked to develop guidelines and levels of care for PICUs. In addition, current statements under development by these organizations regarding admission and discharge criteria for the PICU and regionalization of care recognize the need for establishing standards in these areas. Interfacility transport guidelines also have been formally addressed by the AAP because the transfer of patients requiring specialized care is such a critical step in the process.

A number of EMS-C projects have recognized the importance of the pediatric critical care center as an essential component within the system. Guidelines have been developed and implemented by local EMS agencies in some states to ensure the inclusion of pediatric critical care center standards in the EMS system.

Significant technological advancements have improved the capabilities of pediatric healthcare physicians. They include more sophisticated monitoring techniques, point-of-care microsample testing, ventilatory support devices such as high-frequency oscillators with specific pediatric capabilities, extracorporeal membrane oxygenators, and advanced imaging technologies.

Finally, the emerging importance of managed-care systems has changed the structure of the traditional patient referral system. Close attention to recommended guidelines for pediatric critical care centers will be necessary for the practitioner to ensure that the patient reaches the most appropriate facility, regardless of the type of healthcare coverage. In particular, it must be recognized that the outcomes for the critically ill and injured pediatric patient is improved by the specialized pediatric critical care center.

Definitions of Levels of Receiving Centers

In 1989, the American Medical Association Commission on Emergency Medical Services issued Guidelines for the Categorization of Hospital Emergency Capabilities. One part of these guidelines defines levels of care available to critically ill and injured pediatric patients. Specific requirements for three levels of care are delineated. These guidelines are currently being revisited and revised.

In the AMA guidelines, a Level III receiving facility is defined as a hospital that has the ability to evaluate, stabilize, and transfer seriously ill and injured pediatric patients to higher levels of pediatric care and that should have formalized transfer agreements with those higher-level pediatric care facilities. A Level II receiving facility is a hospital with a pediatric service that is capable of caring for most pediatric patients but has limited pediatric critical care and subspecialty resources. A Level I receiving facility is a center that is capable of providing comprehensive care to critically ill and injured children and has subspecialty pediatric medical and surgical services available at the facility. Finally, some confusion may exist regarding the similarity of terms for facilities. For this chapter, the receiving facility is called the pediatric critical care center, whereas the sending facility is called the referring center.

Although the AMA has not yet completed its revision of these guidelines, the AAP published a revision of "Guidelines for Pediatric Emergency Care Facilities" in 1995 (see Suggested Reading).

The AMA Commission Guidelines provide one system of categorization of levels of care. Other professional and state organizations have addressed categorization as well. The AAP and SCCM published minimal standards for two levels of pediatric critical care: PICUs and pediatric acute care units (PACUs). Some EMS agencies have adopted criteria for pediatric critical care centers and pediatric trauma centers (PTCs) developed by EMS-C coalitions within their states. These centers incorporate many of the minimal standards set by the AAP and SCCM for PICUs. In turn, the PCCCs and PTCs can be considered equivalent to the AMA Commission Level I facilities. This chapter focuses primarily on the pediatric critical care center as the receiving facility.

Because the reproduction of all available standards that have been developed to date is beyond the scope of this book, the reader is referred to the reference documents that identify the specific requirements set forth for pediatric critical care centers. The next section contains a general outline of the essential elements that make up a pediatric critical care center.

The Pediatric Critical Care Center

All pediatric critical care centers must have the following components in place:

1. Administrative organization of the PCCC within the receiving hospital

2. Physician staffing and specialty availability
3. Nursing services and administration
4. Other professional services
5. Emergency department
6. Surgical service and postanesthetic care unit (PACU)
7. Pediatric intensive care unit
8. Special services and resources
9. Support services
10. Policies
11. Continuous quality improvement program
12. Outreach and education programs
13. Transfer agreements
14. Pediatric critical care center equipment supplies and medications for the care of pediatric patients in the emergency department, PICU, and operating room (OR)

Key characteristics that distinguish the PCCC include: institutional recognition of multidisciplinary practice and organization across departments and disciplines, availability of qualified specialists (in-house 24 hours/day as well as on call to the facility), physician and nursing specialists with clearly delineated qualifications based on training and certification, and unit-specific standards (PICU, emergency department, OR) that address the care of critically ill and injured children. Support services such as the clinical laboratory and radiology must be capable of providing pediatric-specific services and expertise.

It is recommended that the PCCC incorporate available standards for emergency departments, as well as the most recent recommendations set forth in "Guidelines and Levels of Care for Pediatric Intensive Care Units" by the AAP and SCCM (see Suggested Reading). Consideration should also be given to the AAP transport guidelines.

Continuous quality-improvement programs should be multidisciplinary and track all critically ill or injured pediatric patients, develop indicators and monitors of patient care, and monitor professional education.

Outreach and Education Programs

The PCCC must ensure that continuing education in pediatric emergency and critical care is provided for its physician, nursing, and allied health personnel. It is also the responsibility of the PCCC to provide outreach education to persons and facilities in the community (such as local EMS personnel, community physicians, nurses, and healthcare personnel) as well as those in its larger referral region. Outreach efforts may be informal (a PCCC specialist speaking at a referring facility's grand rounds) or formal (a contract with a referring facility to provide a certain number of lectures and case reviews to physicians and nurses). The PCCC should also have the resources to provide public education and illness- and injury-prevention education to the public.

Consultation

The PCCC should provide telephone and on-site consultations with physicians, nurses, and other healthcare physicians in the community and outlying areas and with affiliated and referring institutions. Twenty-four-hour availability of these services is essential in assisting with the stabilization and management of critically ill and injured children. These consultations provide a means for deciding on and arranging for the appropriate transfer of patients.

Transfer Criteria

Ideally, each community, primary-care physician and referring facility should identify an appropriate PCCC to receive critically ill and injured pediatric patients. Develop transfer, admission, discharge, and return criteria in conjunction with this process that will facilitate the transfer of patients to higher levels of care, as well as determine when patients may be transferred back to the community hospital. Guidelines for admission to and discharge from PICUs are currently being reviewed by the AAP and SCCM and will be issued jointly in the near future. Interfacility pediatric trauma and critical care consultation and transfer guidelines have also been developed by a number of EMS-C projects and the AAP.

Communication and Coordination of Care

A large number of caregivers, institutions, and agencies take part in the care of critically ill and injured children. The optimal care of these children can be attained only if their care is provided in a coordinated fashion with accurate and timely communication. The care process may begin with an out-of-hospital care physician, continue with a community referring hospital, and end with transfer to a pediatric critical care center (PCCC). Appropriate medical control of the out-of-hospital care phase will ensure that the patient reaches a facility capable of further stabilization. At that point, the referring facility works in conjunction with the PCCC to assess and manage the patient. The consultation process will determine if the patient will require transfer to a higher level of care. The PCCC can assist in stabilizing the patient until the transfer can take place, consult with the referral hospital to determine the appropriate level of transport, and assist in arranging the proper mode of transport. Open communication and cooperation by all participants will ensure that the patient is provided definitive care in a safe, timely, and efficient manner.

Referral Back to the Community Hospital

Many critically ill and injured children are transferred to a geographically distant PCCC for the initial part of their hospitalization. However, during the recovery phase, their care may be appropriately provided at a facility in the community from which they were referred. This option may be preferable for the patient's family and is psychosocially beneficial by enabling the family to spend more time with the patient and the rest of the family. One common obstacle to the back-transfer process is that payers frequently deny payment for the back transport itself, placing this financial burden on the family. The primary-care physician in conjunction with the PCCC can serve as an important advocate for the patient and the family.

Transfer Agreements

Formal transfer agreements should be established by referring community facilities with identified PCCCs. These agreements define the responsibilities of all participating parties, identify mechanisms for initiating transfer, and provide for the return of patients to the community hospital. A community hospital may have transfer agreements with more than one PCCC. A model pediatric interfacility transfer agreement appears in the Appendix at the end of this chapter.

Summary

Pediatric critical care centers are an important link in the chain of survival for critically ill and injured children. They provide highly specialized emergency critical care and pediatric medical and surgical subspecialty support to improve outcomes. These referral centers also serve as sources for consultation and education for the community, and formal links should be made between community practitioners and hospitals and the referral centers.

Suggested Reading

American Medical Association Commission on Emergency Medical Services. Pediatric emergencies: an excerpt from "Guidelines for the Categorization of Hospital Emergency Capabilities." *Pediatrics.* 1990;85:879–887

American Academy of Pediatrics Committee on Hospital Care, American College of Critical Care Medicine, and Pediatric Section of the Society of Critical Care Medicine. Guidelines for developing admission and discharge policies for the pediatric intensive care unit. *Pediatrics.* 1999;103:840–842

American Academy of Pediatrics Committee on Hospital Care and Pediatric Section of the Society of Critical Care Medicine. Guidelines and levels of care for pediatric intensive care units. *Pediatrics.* 1993;92:166–175, *Crit Care Med.* 1993;21:1077–1086

American Academy of Pediatrics Committee on Pediatric Emergency Medicine. Guidelines for pediatric emergency care facilities. *Pediatrics.* 1995;96:526–537

American Academy of Pediatrics Committee on Pediatric Emergency Medicine, American College of Critical Care Medicine, and Pediatric Section of the Society of Critical Care Medicine. Consensus report for regionalization of care for critically ill or injured children. *Pediatrics.* 2000;105:152–155

Henderson DP, Seidel JS, eds. *Emergency Medical Services for Children: Development and Integration of Pediatric Emergency Care into EMS Systems.* U.S. Department of Health and Human Services, Health Resources and Services Administration. Los Angeles, CA: California State Department of Health; 1991

Pediatric Emergency Medical Services Advisory Board. *A Plan for Regionalization: Emergency Medical Services for Children In Oregon and Southwest Washington.* Portland, OR: Health Division, Oregon Department of Human Resources; 1988: Appendix Cf

Pettigrew AH, Moody RR. Pediatric critical care systems. In: Dieckmann RA, ed. *Pediatric Emergency Care Systems Planning and Management.* Baltimore, MD: Williams & Wilkins; 1992:279–294

State of California Emergency Medical Services Authority. Emergency Medical Services Authority. State of California Emergency Medical Services for Children. Final report. Sacramento, CA, November 1994

State of California Emergency Medical Services Authority. *Interfacility and Specialized Centers Guidelines.* U.S. Department of Health and Human Services, Health Resources and Services Administration. Sacramento, CA; 1994

Appendix: Model Pediatric Interfacility Transfer Agreement

AGREEMENT

This AGREEMENT is made between SPECIALIZED REFERRAL CENTER (CENTER)* located at

_____

and HOSPITAL located at

_____

hence forth referred to as HOSPITAL or referring hospital.

This Agreement serves as documentation of the arrangements, policies, and procedures governing the transfer of critically ill and/or injured pediatric patients (...Add other types of patients or services, if desired...) between the above named institutions in order to facilitate timely transfer, continuity of care, and appropriate transport for these patients.

THE CENTER AND HOSPITAL DO MUTUALLY AGREE AS FOLLOWS:

1. HOSPITAL recognizes that on certain occasions pediatric patients require specialized care and services beyond the scope of services available at HOSPITAL and that optimal care of these children requires transfer from the ED or inpatient services to centers with specialized pediatric critical care or pediatric trauma services.

---

* Specialized referral centers for pediatric critical care and/or pediatric trauma care, may include: (1) Pediatric Critical Care Center(s), (2) Pediatric Trauma Centers(s), or (3) General Trauma Center(s), Burn Center(s), etc.

2. The medical staff and hospital administration of HOSPI-
   TAL have identified the CENTER as a pediatric critical
   care center with specialized staff and facilities for terti-
   ary-level care of critically ill and/or injured children.
3. The CENTER agrees to maintain a regional (Tertiary) (1)
   Pediatric Critical Care Center, (2) Pediatric Trauma Center,
   or (3) General Trauma Center that is equipped and staffed
   to provide a full range of pediatric medical and surgical
   services for critically ill pediatric patients and/or pediatric
   trauma patients in accordance with currently published
   Pediatric Intensive Care Unit standards, or applicable
   State and local EMS Agency standards for Pediatric Critical Care Centers, Pediatric Trauma Centers, or General
   Trauma Centers.
4. The CENTER agrees to accept transfers of critically ill
   and injured pediatric patients from HOSPITAL, if beds,
   personnel, and appropriate services are available, if the
   transfer has been approved by the receiving physician,
   and if the transfer is consistent with current patient
   transfer laws.
5. Pursuant to CCS requirements for regional (tertiary) level
   approval and State Trauma System regulations, CENTERS
   will provide 24-hour telephone consultation services, 24-
   hour pediatric transport services, and educational programs related to pediatric emergency, critical care, and/or
   trauma care that can be made available to community
   health professionals involved in such care.
6. HOSPITAL and CENTER recognize the privilege of an
   attending physician and the right of the patient, or the
   patient through a relative or guardian, to request transfer
   to an alternate facility.

Indications for Pediatric Transfers

7. The referring physician has examined the patient, documented the patient's condition, and has determined that
   the patient requires a higher level of care than provided
   at HOSPITAL or requires specialized services provided at
   the CENTER.
8. The referring physician has evaluated the patient and
   has determined that the transport is compatible with the

patient's condition and is in the best interests of the patient's medical care.

Transfer Arrangements

9. Requests for consultation or transport team support and patient transfer can be generated by telephone to:
    (List appropriate telephone numbers for pediatric critical care, trauma, transport, and other services, as appropriate.)

10. When it appears that a pediatric patient requires specialized services or medical care beyond the scope of services provided at HOSPITAL, the referring physician shall contact an appropriate specialist at the CENTER to obtain consultation. The referring physician in conjunction with the CENTER consultant shall be responsible for determining the need for admission to the CENTER. The consent of appropriately authorized staff at the CENTER to receive the patient shall be obtained prior to the patient's release from HOSPITAL and shall be documented in the patient's medical record.

11. Transfer arrangements will be made by mutual consent of the referring and consulting physician. It shall be the responsibility of the physician to whom the patient is transferred to arrange the admission of the patient to the CENTER. If the CENTER is unable to accept the patient because of lack of physical or professional resources, the CENTER personnel will assist the referring hospital in locating an alternative center for patient placement.

12. The referring physician, in consultation with the receiving physician, shall determine the method of transport to be used. The CENTER may, at its option, provide a specially trained pediatric transport team. The team shall be in attendance during the entire transport.

13. To the extent possible, patients will be stabilized prior to transfer and treatment initiated to ensure that the transfer will not, within reasonable medical probability, result in harm to the patient or jeopardize survival. Responsibility for the stabilization and care of patients prior to and during transport should be specified.

14. The referring hospital shall be responsible for informing the patient, patient's parent(s), legal guardian, or other

relatives of the transfer process and for obtaining any release to effect the transfer. The referring hospital shall use its best efforts to arrange for the parent(s) or guardian to be present at the time of transport and provide them with all necessary information about the transport to the receiving hospital.

15. The referring hospital shall be responsible for the transfer or other appropriate disposition of any personal belongings of the patient.

Records and Transmission of Information

16. Subject to federal and state laws regarding consents of minors for medical care and confidentiality of medical information, the referring hospital shall send with the patient, or arrange to be immediately transmitted (via FAX), at the time of transfer the necessary documents and completed forms containing the medical, social, and/or other information necessary to ensure continuity of care of the patient. Such documentation shall include at least the following:
    a. Identification of the patient
    b. Diagnosis
    c. Copies of the relevant portions of the patient's medical record (including medical, nursing, dietary, laboratory, X-rays, and medication records)
    d. Phone numbers to obtain results of laboratory values and other tests pending at the time of transport
    e.. Relevant transport forms
    f. Copy of signed consent for transport of a minor

17. Subject to limitations regarding confidentiality, the CENTER shall provide information on the patient's diagnosis, condition, treatment, prognosis, and any complications to the referring physician during the time that the patient is hospitalized at the CENTER and upon discharge or transfer from the CENTER.

Return of Patient to Referring Hospital

18. When the patient's physician at the CENTER determines that the patient is medically fit for return to the referring hospital, that physician should contact an appropriate physician at the referring hospital to arrange for the

return of the patient. The CENTER shall send with the patient at the time of transfer the necessary documents and forms containing the medical, social, and/or other information necessary to ensure continuity of care of the patient. The CENTER shall be responsible for informing the patient, patient's parent(s), or legal guardian of the transfer process and for obtaining any releases required for the transfer or the appropriate disposition of any personal effects of the patient. The CENTER will be responsible for arranging patient transport to referring hospital.

19. The return transfer of pediatric patient for continued care upon completion of the treatment at the CENTER will be made by mutual agreement.

Charges for Services

20. Charges for services performed by either institution shall be made and collected by the institution in accordance with its regular policies and procedures. Unless special arrangements have been made to the contrary, the transfer of a patient from one institution to the other shall not be construed as imposing any financial liability by one institution on the other. The parties shall cooperate with each other in the exchange of information about financial responsibility for the services rendered by them to patients who are transferred to the CENTER.

Authority of Governing Bodies

21. The Governing Body of each institution shall have exclusive control of its policies, management, assets, and affairs, and neither shall incur any responsibility by virtue of this Agreement for any debts or other financial obligations incurred by the other. Further, nothing in this Agreement shall be construed as limiting the rights of either institution to contract with any other facility on a limited or general basis.

Term of Agreement

22. The term of this Agreement shall commence on _____ and shall continue in full force and effect until _____. Either institution may terminate this Agreement at any time upon giving the other written notice not less than thirty (30) days in

advance of the termination date. However, should either institution fail to maintain its license or certification, this Agreement shall automatically terminate as of the date of termination of the license or certification.

Indemnification

23. The parties agree to indemnify, defend, and hold one another, their officers, agents, and employees harmless from and against any and all liability, loss, expense, attorney's fees, or claims for injury or damages arising out of their performance of this Agreement, but only in proportion to and to the extent such liability, loss, expense, attorney's fees, or claims for injury or damages are caused by or result from the negligent or intentional act or omission of the indemnifying party.

Compliance with Laws and Regulations

24. This Agreement is entered into and shall be performed by both parties in compliance with local, state, and federal laws, rules, regulations, and guidelines, including COBRA and OBRA.

Insurance Provisions

25. The parties hereto warrant they shall obtain and maintain during the term hereof, at their own sole cost and expense, insurance or a program of self-insurance covering their activities in performance hereof.

General Provisions

26. This Agreement constitutes the entire understanding of the parties hereto with respect to the matters discussed herein and supersedes any and all written or oral agreements, representations, or understandings, whether made by the parties or others purportedly on behalf of one of the parties. No changes, amendments, or alterations of this Agreement shall be effective, unless made in writing and signed by both parties.

27. It is not the intention of either party that any person or entity be a third party beneficiary of this Agreement.

28. Neither party may assign, sell, or otherwise transfer this Agreement, or any interest in it, without the express prior written approval of the other.

29. Any notice required or permitted by this Agreement shall

be effective and shall be deemed delivered five (5) business days after placing it in the mail, by certified mail, return receipt requested, postage prepaid, or upon personal delivery as follows:

To: Administrator
CENTER Address

To: Administrator
HOSPITAL Address

IN WITNESS WHEREOF, the parties have executed this Agreement on the date written below.

HOSPITAL (Name and Address)   CENTER (Name and Address)

_____   _____

_____   _____

Chief Executive Officer   Chief Executive Officer

Name _____   Name _____

Title _____   Title _____

Date _____   Date _____

_____   _____

Chief of Medical Staff   Medical Director of PICU

_____   _____

Chief of Pediatrics   Chief of Pediatrics

                               _____

                               Chief of Trauma Service

_____   _____

Chief of Emergency
Medicine

Medical Director of
Emergency Dept.

Death of a Child

Introduction

The most painful event imaginable for a family is the death of their child. Even when parents are somewhat prepared for the possibility of the child's death, as with chronic illness, the loss is totally devastating—parents not only lose the joy and wonder of the child as a person, but must relinquish their hopes and dreams for the child as well. The death of a child also has a ripple effect in the community of care surrounding the child; extended family, friends, caretakers, and health professionals are all affected. Coping effectively with families after this tragic event can be both painful and rewarding.

Most child deaths in the early years are from SIDS, prematurity, congenital anomalies, and infections. When children are able to walk, traumatic injury—falls, motor vehicle injuries, and drowning—becomes a more common cause of death. Motor vehicle deaths are the most common cause in the teenage years. Most healthcare physicians readily admit that caring for critically ill and injured children is stressful and that helping a family cope with the death of a child is an intense emotional experience. Primary-care physicians have to handle their own reactions to the death, as well as the professional matters that death entails, and often they have little preparation for this task. Because the focus of most medical education and training is on alleviating pain and curing illness, little attention is given to learning about death and dying.

When a child dies in an acute-care setting, it is common for physicians to find themselves in the difficult position of providing both the technical expertise necessary for the care of an ill or injured child and the emotional support necessary for the family after the child's death. Because the death of a child is a rare event, professionals may be in need of comfort themselves in coping with the death. An additional complication may be the perception of guilt or failure on the part of the physician in the death of the child, regardless of the reality of the situation. Although each child's death is unique, there are also many common features in the grieving process. Research in this area has shown that both training and experience in working with families after the death of a child increase the comfort level of physicians in providing information to families and helping them through the early stages of grief. Families who have experienced the death of a child are an excellent source of information on what interventions are helpful in this process.

Parents

There are several models for conceptualizing the grieving process; the most commonly known is the sequence of emotional stages described by Elizabeth Kübler-Ross: denial, anger, bargaining, depression, and acceptance. Although this model provides a general framework for understanding bereavement, the specific emotional stages are not necessarily experienced by all persons and may not evolve consecutively. In the acute-care setting, professionals often witness emotions such as denial, anger, bargaining, and depression of families but rarely witness acceptance, which requires substantial processing over time. Because of the physician's concern for the family, there is often hope for rapid progression to the acceptance stage, even in the acute-care setting. The process of grieving, however, is unique to each person, and professional intervention requires the assurance of a supportive, nonjudgmental atmosphere where families feel safe in experiencing their pain and loss in their own way and in their own time.

Many families have been asked what was helpful to them after the death of a family member; the answers obtained are very consistent. Initially, they would like to have:

- privacy
- access to information about the patient's condition and to be kept up to date
- comfort measures including adequate seating, tissues, and

access to a telephone
• an identifiable person to serve as liaison

All of these objectives are important and should be included in the planning process in preparing for helping families with the death of a child in an acute-care setting.

Privacy and Comfort

Not all facilities are able to provide a private room for the family; nevertheless a private room should be a priority. Any location where the family can remain out of direct public view can be used. Families should also have comfortable seating, as well as a telephone, tissues, and a bathroom nearby. Provide coffee, tea, or water to help establish a comforting structure for the family. If the wait is long, the staff should provide food for the family.

Family Presence

A dying child may be aware of much that goes on, even when he or she is unresponsive; so talking to the child and ensuring the child's comfort, privacy, and modesty should be a part of caring for the child. It is easy to get caught up in performing procedures and giving medications, forgetting that the child is a person and may be aware that he or she is dying. Allowing the family to be present during a child's resuscitation is a controversial issue. Parents who have been allowed into the resuscitation room before the death of a family member overwhelmingly cite the importance of this opportunity to say good-bye and describe their conviction that they were of some help to the deceased during that time. This issue is difficult, however, because many staff members are uncomfortable in the presence of the family, fearing that the family will make judgments or prove to be unable to handle the situation.

If the family is allowed to be present during resuscitation, a staff member must take responsibility for staying with them, explaining the procedures, and assisting them in leaving the treatment room. It is not advisable for the family to be present throughout the entire resuscitative effort, but holding a dying child's hand, talking to the child, or touching a foot may give comfort to the child. It also acknowledges the reality of the situation and provides an entry into the grieving process.

Informing the Family

If there will be a waiting period for the family, a designated staff person should serve as liaison, checking back with the family throughout and providing updated information. For an anxious family, 5 minutes can be an interminably long wait for information. The hospital chaplain is often available to assist the family and skilled in dealing with the grieving process. The family should also be offered the presence of religious support if they wish it—the liaison should contact the appropriate religious institution (a list should be available for use in such an emergency). If resuscitation is under way, give the family as much information as possible about the child's condition, without raising false hopes. Observe the family's reaction to be sure that the seriousness of the situation is understood; remember that telling a family that the child is not breathing and does not have a pulse may not necessarily be interpreted by the family as grave because of the way resuscitation is portrayed in the media.

Physicians must assume responsibility for informing the family of the death of a child. Inform the family immediately after the death is pronounced, however difficult the task. When informing the family about the child's condition, a team approach is most effective. The team may include a nurse, a social worker, and a pastor, depending on the situation and availability of personnel and the needs of the family. The family may have questions about the death or of what will happen next; having a professional stay with them for support after they have been informed of the death is essential.

When informing the family of the death, the message should be unequivocal: the word "dead" or "died" must be used. Use of terms such as "passed away" or statements such as "we were unable to resuscitate your child" may be misinterpreted, because of the high level of denial on the family's part. There is little or no need at this point to explain what treatments were used or other medical facts unless the family asks questions. Support after the announcement of the death must be guided by the family's needs. The most important information is that the child has died, and the family must be informed of that fact without delay. Announcement of the child's death may be followed (or preceded) with a simple statement such as "I am so sorry," expressing your concern for the family and respect for their pain. Resist the impulse to say, "I understand" or "I know how you feel," however, even when you have experienced a similar event, because the family is truly alone in experiencing the loss of their child and cannot imagine how any other person's experiences could relate to theirs.

Emotional Responses

When the family has been informed of the child's death, the grieving process may take many forms. The family may appear calm, agitated, frantic, confused, angry, despairing, in full denial, immobilized, or in total collapse. Allow the family to express their emotions, without judgment. Different people and different cultures have widely varying methods of emotional expression. Anger may be expressed against caregivers, against other family members, and against God. Men are more likely than women to express grief in physical activity or violence, by hitting a wall, throwing a chair, or by loud verbal abuse. Family members may completely deny the child's death initially with statements such as, "Look, he's breathing!" Remember that denial is powerful and protective at this point and will eventually go away. Only when denial persists over a period of days or weeks is there cause for concern.

Questions

Family members may have many questions, some spoken, some left unasked. The most common questions are:

- *"Was my child in pain?"* If the child was unconscious throughout, it is fairly easy to answer this question with a simple "No." If the child was crying, screaming, or combative, the easiest answer may be to say quite truthfully, "It is hard to know what children experience in these conditions."
- *"How did this happen?"* Usually this question is not meant literally, but is an attempt to reconstruct the incident to determine what could have been done differently.

  Parents invariably assume some degree of responsibility for their child's death, even when it is clear that they were not directly responsible. If the family does not bring up the issue of guilt, it may be helpful to bring it up yourself by saying, "Many times, family members feel responsible in some way for their child's death. Are you feeling that?" If a family actually has had some part in the child's death through inattention or neglect, this fact is something that will have to be dealt with at some point, and bringing it up only gives permission for them to begin processing the issue.

- *"Why did this happen?"* This is a philosophical question; the answer will come to the family at a much later time. It is important not to offer an answer based on your own religious or philosophical framework, because that answer may not be appropriate for the family. The simplest answer is, "I wish I had an answer for you." Such a statement assures the family that you are on their side, without providing an answer that may not fit their belief system.

- *"What do we do now?"* When a family asks this question, they are usually concretely asking what will happen in the next few minutes or hours.

    The answer will depend on the setting and situation. In most acute-care settings, the family can be allowed to view or hold the child or both. You may want to wait awhile, perhaps until after the family has held the child, to deal with such matters as the need for an autopsy, mortuary arrangements, and the possibility of organ donation, depending on the circumstances.

Viewing the Body

When a death occurs in an acute-care setting, the parent(s) should be provided with an opportunity to see, touch, and hold the dead child. Although it is rare for a parent to forgo this opportunity, each parent should be asked individually. Parents may have mixed feelings, and one parent may try to protect or coerce the other. The staff liaison should tell the family how the child looks and instruct them in what is allowed—removing tubes, for instance, is usually not permissible when a coroner's autopsy will be performed. Holding the child may take several hours, so the child may have to be moved to an out-of-the-way location before the family is brought in.

The family may want to be alone with the child; if this is feasible, a staff member should check with them periodically, because the family may feel awkward in asking to leave. When the family is ready to leave, a staff member should stay with the child, because many parents feel that their child should not be left alone in the room.

Closing

Before the family leaves, several important matters must be addressed: autopsy permission, organ donation, and mortuary selection. Permission for autopsy is not necessary, because all unexpected deaths in the emergency department must be reported to the coroner or medical examiner. The exception to this rule applies to a child who has had a chronic illness and there is a physician willing to sign the death certificate. The coroner or medical examiner in many states will decide the need for an autopsy.

Although health professionals are often uncomfortable with addressing the question of organ donation, families are often grateful that something positive results from their child's death. Remember that some religions and cultures do not approve of organ transplant, and some families are very uncomfortable with the idea; this question should be carefully approached. Many regional procurement agencies are willing to come and talk with the family directly and are very experienced in addressing this matter with families. Remember that some states have laws mandating requests for organ donation. Know your states statutes on this subject.

In some facilities, social workers or clergy are available to assist in the choice of a mortuary, which must be made within hours of the death. Advance preparation for handling the death of a child in an acute-care facility should include having a handout for families that contains a list of mortuaries and the cost of funeral arrangements at each one clearly laid out. Most parents have not considered the possibility of the death of a child and have no idea where to turn. Written materials provide opportunities for careful consideration, as well as the inclusion of relatives and friends in making the decision.

In addition to the essential procedures and paperwork heretofore described, several interventions are a part of bereavement protocols at some hospitals. They may not be appropriate for all facilities but are listed here because they have been found to be helpful to families:

1. Providing the family with a photograph of the deceased. This is done most frequently if a child is stillborn, but it has been done for other children. Parents have considered the photograph to be a way of remembering the child, especially when the child is taken directly to a mortuary after the death.
2. Cutting off a lock of hair to give to the family. This gives a family a tactile remembrance of the child.
3. Taking an imprint of the child's hand or foot in plaster. There are many kits available to do this rapidly, and families have found this to be comforting.
4. Arranging for the family to receive a baptismal or other written remembrance from clergy who attend to the family. This becomes a treasured remembrance for the family.
5. Sending a card or brief personal note to the family. A telephone call may be awkward and the timing may be difficult, whereas a written note can show concern for the family and is less intrusive. Some healthcare physicians may choose to attend the funeral when the child and family are long-term patients.

These interventions may be very helpful to families, but their use must be guided by each family's needs, rather than being included routinely in bereavement protocols.

Siblings

Families may ask you about how to handle questions from siblings and whether siblings should attend the funeral. Most experts agree that a basic awareness of death develops at about 3 years of age, so the family must make some careful decisions about how the family will approach the matter with siblings. Children younger than 3 may be able to stay at home with relatives during the funeral, but, at 4 or 5 years of age, as children become able to make rational choices, they may want to decide for themselves whether they want to attend. Whatever the family decides about funeral attendance, there may be more harm in withholding information from siblings and attempting to insulate them than there is in including them in the family grieving process.

Informing the Primary-Care Physician

Inform the primary-care physician about the death of the child as soon as possible. Include the circumstances of the incident, the details of the resuscitation, and any pertinent information about the family and autopsy.

Advanced Preparation for Death of a Child

Advance planning can facilitate coping with the death of a child. The most important advanced preparations are shown in Table 14. Some institutions have a packet of all necessary forms, resources, and other pertinent materials to be used in the event of a death.

Table 14.

Advanced Preparation for Death of a Child

- Identification of staff members willing to assist families in the event of the death of a child. Such staff members may include social workers, nurses, aides, and ancillary staff who may be available when a death occurs.
- Location of a private area for families of critically ill or injured children. Even when a private room is not available, plans should be made to use a specific area away from public view.
- Education of staff in coping with families after the death of a child. Such education should be periodically updated if the interval between deaths is lengthy. Include information about handling deaths in orientation programs.
- Written protocols for handling the death of a child, including a checklist of items such as: organ donation, notification of coroner, autopsy, death certificate, referrals, contact person, and list of mortuaries.
- Development and regular updating of a list of clergy from the most common religious organizations. Clergy should be contacted in advance to ask about availability in an emergency.
- Planning for critical incident stress management. When there is a death of a staff member or a member of his or her family, when there are multiple deaths, or when the death of a child is particularly tragic or unusual, critical incident stress defusing or debriefing should be made available.

Summary

As the family prepares to leave, any written materials or referrals may be offered. The family's questions and concerns should be the guide for providing them. Attempts to reassure the family at this point or to give information about the grieving process have been noted to be useless, because the family is simply trying to manage to get through the next few hours. Remember that you cannot make family members feel better; you can only provide a supportive atmosphere in which they can grieve. Your essential role is to make sure that all procedures are carried out as smoothly as possible and that all of the family's needs and concerns are addressed. Although helping a family through this painful experience can be emotionally draining, there are many rewards in providing caring, competent care for them at this difficult time in their lives, which can affect the family system for many years to come. A review of the general rules for coping with the death of a child can be found in the Appendix at the end of this chapter.

Suggested Reading

Becker E. *The Denial of Death*. New York, NY: Free Press; 1973

Cohen GJ. Children dead on arrival: predictors of short-term family follow-up. *Am J Emerg Med.*1984;2:315–320

daSilva GC. Awareness of Hispanic cultural issues in the health care setting. *Childrens Health Care.* 1984;13:4–10

Feifel H. *The Meaning of Death*. New York: McGraw-Hill, 1959

Fischhoff J, O'Brien N. After the child dies. *J Pediatr.* 1976;88:140–146

Frader JE, Sargent J. Sudden death or catastrophic illness: family considerations. In: Fleisher GR, Ludwig S, eds. *Textbook of Pediatric Emergency Medicine*. 3rd ed. Baltimore, MD: Williams & Wilkins; 1988:1164–1173

Leopold RL, Dillon H. Psycho-anatomy of a disaster: a long-term study of post-traumatic neuroses in survivors of a marine explosion. *Am J Psychiatry.* 1963;119:913–921

Linderman E. Symptomatology and management of acute grief. *Am J Psychiatry.* 1944;101:141–148

Meares RA. On saying good-bye before death. *JAMA.* 1981;246: 1227–1229

Segal S, Fletcher M, Meekison WG. Survey of bereaved parents. *CMAJ*. 1986;134:38–42

Williams M. Use of a concluding process to assist grieving families. *J Emerg Nurs*. 1984;10:254–258

Yalom ID. *Existential Psychotherapy*. New York, NY: Basic Books; 1980

Appendix: General Rules for Coping with the Death of a Child

On Initial Contact
- Give accurate information
- Offer whatever privacy you can
- Accommodate physical needs: bathroom, water, tissues
- Offer religious support, including baptism and last rites

Informing the Family of the Child's Death
- Inform the family immediately; give a brief explanation if asked
- Sit down with family
- Use the word "death" or "died"
- Address the matters of pain and guilt
- Allow the family to express emotions, unjudgmentally
- Allow time for questions

Holding, Staying with the Child
- Ask each family member separately if he or she wants to be with the child
- Tell the family about tubes, wires, and so forth, before the family enters the room
- Stay with the family briefly; make sure that someone will check back
- Allow family members as much time as they need for closure, but assure them that they can leave when they wish
- A staff member should stay in the room with the child when the family leaves

Closing Issues
- Organ donation
- Explain about coroner and autopsy

- Provide information about mortuaries
- Complete paperwork: release of the body, death certificate, permission for autopsy

Most Common Questions

- Most common (often unstated): Was it my/our fault in some way?
- Was there pain?
- Why? (Do not attempt to answer this question.)
- What happens now (in the next few minutes, hours)?
- What should I/we tell siblings?
- Should young children attend funeral?

DO

- Tell the family how sorry you are.
- Tell family whom they can call if they have questions later.
- Give written instructions and referrals.
- If the family desires a follow-up visit to give them additional information, schedule the visit.

DON'T

- Do not say, "I know how you feel."
- Do not say, "You have other children" or "You can have other children."
- Do not attempt to answer the question, "Why?"
- Do not try to tell family that they will feel better in time.

Part IV

Community Preparation

The individual practitioner and hospital are part of the community. The components of EMS-C in the community include, among others, out-of-hospital services, the care of children with special health-care needs, and the care of children through the implementation of organized emergency systems in the event of a disaster. The preparation of the community is a major

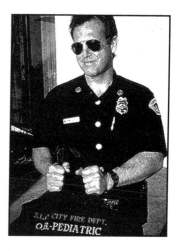

undertaking, which requires skills in advocacy and coalition building.

Chapter 14

Out-of-Hospital Care
of Pediatric Patients

Important Considerations About Out-of-Hospital Care

1. Know your EMS system and the types of physicians.
2. Know the particulars of your community emergency response number.
3. Make sure that transport vehicles have pediatric equipment and supplies.

Introduction

Although the history of the modern ambulance begins in Napoleon's time, the true development of emergency medical services (EMS) began in earnest in 1966, when a report titled Accidental Death and Disability: The Neglected Disease of Modern Society [published by the National Academy of Sciences (NAS) and the National Research Council (NRC)] documented the deficiencies of the EMS systems of that time.

Knowledge gained in the Korean and Vietnam Wars demonstrated that rapid triage, transport, and treatment to a field hospital of the seriously injured soldier resulted in improved care. At the same time in Northern Ireland, mobile intensive care units staffed by physicians demonstrated improved survival in patients with cardiac emergencies. In 1970, the NAS and the NRC made recommendations on ways to improve emergency medical care, including increased attention to injury prevention, standards and regulations for ambulance services, adoption of ways to coordinate ambulance services with hospitals, a single emergency access number, delineation of radio-frequency channels and equipment to provide communication between ambulance and emergency department, and development of a mechanism for inspection, categorization, and accreditation of emergency departments. The concept of a "systems" approach came in 1973 with the federal program authorized by the Emergency Medical Services Systems (EMSS) Act. The act promoted the development of regional systems built around the key components as listed in Table 15.

Table 15.

Key Components of EMS

Personnel
Training
Communication
Transportation
Medical facilities
Critical care units
Public safety agencies
Access to care
Patient transfer
Coordinated patient record keeping
Public information and education
Review and evaluation
Disaster linkage
Mutual aid
Consumer participation

Funding from federal and private sources led to substantial improvements in EMS systems, but children were not often beneficiaries of these changes. The incorporation of children's needs into the EMS system began slowly in the late 1970s but gained momentum in the 1980s with the development of pediatric basic and advanced life support courses and the authorization of federal funding for Emergency Medical Services for Children (EMS-C) in 1984.

Although all of the components of an EMS system will not be covered in this chapter, several of them will be described as a basis for understanding of what makes up an EMS system.

Types of EMS Systems

Although the specific municipal agency that manages the EMS system varies throughout the United States, there are several common approaches: a fire department alone (provides both fire and EMS, with cross-trained personnel or dedicated EMS personnel), a fire department with a private physician, a private EMS physician, or as a third service, separate from police and fire departments.

Personnel and Training

There are four levels of providers, but not all states use every level.

First Responder. A person, often a law-enforcement officer, firefighter, lifeguard, or forest ranger, among others, who can provide extrication, airway clearance, cardiopulmonary resuscitation (CPR), hemorrhage control, bandaging, splinting, and normal delivery of newborns. The focus of the 40- to 60-hour course is to provide initial stabilization until arrival of an EMS unit.

Emergency Medical Technician-Basic (EMT-B often called an *EMT*). A basic life-support (BLS) provider who is able to evaluate the severity of a medical condition, provide interventions, and transport a patient to the hospital. Skills learned in the new 110-hour course include all interventions of a first responder plus on-scene triage, patient assessment, oxygen administration, assisted ventilation (bag-valve-mask), spinal immobilization, pneumatic antishock garment administration, and oral glucose and activated charcoal administration (with medical direction only). In addition, there is a new component of patient-assisted medication delivery of newborns (to be given only with medical direction). Medications used at this level include epinephrine auto-injector (EpiPen), prescribed inhalers (for asthma), and sublingual nitroglycerin. Despite an expanded didactic pediatric curriculum, only 10 of the 110 hours are spent on pediatric and newborn topics. An optional advanced airway/intubation module also is available, but its use so far is not widespread (and is based on medical-direction decisions).

Emergency Medical Technician-Intermediate (EMT-I). An advanced EMT who has additional training to develop skills such as the use of an automatic external defibrillator (AED; this physician is often called an EMT-D), the initiation of vascular access, the administration of additional medications and intravascular fluids, and the use of an esophageal obturator airway.

Emergency Medical Technician-Paramedic (EMT-P). A paramedic is an advanced life support (ALS) provider who has taken a 400-hour (minimum) course that teaches the skills required at the levels of EMT-B, EMT-D, and EMT-I plus advanced resuscitation procedures. Many courses are much longer than 400 hours, amounting to a range of 1000 to 2000 hours of education that includes classroom (didactic) plus clinical time (spent in emergency departments and intensive care units). (Although the national curriculum is undergoing revision at the present time, the basic skills taught will remain the same, with a slight increase in time spent on pediatric topics.) The skills required for paramedics include rhythm disturbance recognition, synchronized cardioversion, defibrillation, advanced airway management including intubation, and peripheral vascular access. Optimal procedures such as cricothyroidotomy, needle chest decompression, and vascular access through a central vein or intraosseous route are determined by state law and local scope of practice. Paramedics are able to diagnose and treat problems such as anaphylaxis, respiratory distress (asthma versus pulmonary edema), chest pain, eclampsia, shock, seizures, poisoning, and altered level of consciousness (due to drug overdose, hypoglycemia).

Basic Life Support Services (BLS ambulance). Implies that either a first responder, an EMT-B, or two EMT-Bs are providing care.

Advanced Life Support Services (ALS ambulance). Implies that at least one provider is a paramedic, although in many systems both providers are paramedics.

Medical Dispatch

Before an ambulance can be dispatched, the call for help must be received. This is the point at which communications fit into the system. Having one number (such as 911) is the ideal way to access the EMS system, but it is the person who answers the calls who actually assigns priority to them. This person, the emergency medical dispatcher, must be able to obtain the information from the caller, triage calls, determine what type of unit to send (this is especially true in a two-tiered system, described later in this section), give information to responding units, and, in some systems, provide prearrival medical care instructions by telephone before the arrival of the EMS unit. In large cities, these responsibilities may be handled by several people in various ways: in a horizontal configuration, one dispatcher gets the call and another sends the ambulance; in a vertical configuration, one person does all jobs for a given area. Specific training is required for this job as well, usually from 25 to 40 hours. Besides having excellent communication skills, many dispatchers have some EMS background, such as EMT-B training.

Another factor in the dispatch system is the type of EMS system: one tiered or two-tiered. A tiered response requires the availability of one or more types of response vehicles or level of physician or both. In a one-tiered system, only BLS or ALS services respond to each call, whereas a two-tiered system provides a combination of BLS and ALS services and may even include a special response unit (which may not be able to transport the patient) on ambulance calls. In some systems, a BLS and an ALS unit respond to all calls.

Medical Direction

Despite the fact that physicians are rarely seen "in the field," out-of hospital medical care is being overseen by a licensed physician (medical direction or oversight). Although this position is usually held by an emergency medicine physician, it could be held by almost any physician who has an interest in EMS and is dedicated to it. Advanced out-of-hospital care providers perform their duties under the authorization of a system's medical director. Although BLS providers have not had such oversight in the past, with the new curriculum and the National Highway Traffic Safety Administration (NHTSA) document titled "EMS Agenda for the Future," more formal oversight is being sought for all EMS systems, including BLS providers.

Medical direction includes the direction of the EMS system and its providers and is accomplished in several ways. Indirect medical direction (off-line) consists of administrative activities that keep the system functioning smoothly. These administrative activities include personnel selection and retention, quality management and improvement, training and education of providers, developing treatment and transport protocols, conforming to equipment and medication standards, developing a medical direction plan, developing disaster and hazardous materials management plans, budgeting, and billing. Despite the fact that this mainly administrative work is both prospective (training, protocols, system plan) and retrospective (review of ambulance responses, quality improvement), behind the scenes, it is still ultimately responsible for the overall quality of care delivered by the EMS system.

One of the pediatric areas under the jurisdiction of the medical director (if not mandated by state minimal equipment guidelines) is to oversee the type of pediatric equipment and supplies carried in the ambulance, as recently recommended by a National Pediatric Task Force (see Tables 16 and 17). Another area is the number of hours of continuing education, specifically pediatric topics (usually, the state sets a minimal number of hours, with no pediatrics specified; however, local EMS agencies can set their own standards above the state minimum).

Direct (on-line or immediate) medical direction refers to the direction of the out-of-hospital personnel by medical personnel. There is direct communication by radio, by telephone, or on the scene between the physician or physician surrogate (often a specially trained mobile intensive care nurse or paramedic) and the provider (acting as a physician extender) while in the field. In most cases, the out-of-hospital personnel work from a set of guidelines or protocols predetermined by the medical director (off-line medical direction). These guidelines are usually diagnosis or diagnostic category based, such as chest pain, respiratory distress, ventricular tachycardia, altered level of consciousness, and so forth. These guidelines must specify at

Table 16.

BLS Ambulance Pediatric Supplies and Equipment

Essential

Oropharyngeal airways, infant, child, and adult (size 00–5)
Self-inflating resuscitation bag, child and adult size[1]
Masks for bag-valve-mask device, infant, child, and adult[2]
Oxygen masks, infant, child, and adult
Non-rebreathing mask, pediatric and adult
Stethoscope
Backboard
Cervical immobilization device[3]

continued

Table 16. *(continued)*

Blood pressure cuff, infant, child, and adult
Portable suction unit with a regulator
Suction catheters, tonsil tip and 6F–14F
Extremity splints, pediatric sizes
Bulb syringe
Obstetric pack
Thermal blanket[4]
Water soluble lubricant

Desirable

Infant car seat[5]
Nasopharyngeal airways (sizes 18F–34F, or 4.5–8.5 mm)[6]
Glasgow Coma Score reference
Pediatric Trauma Score reference
Small stuffed toy

• •

[1] A self-inflating resuscitation bag should be self-refilling, have an oxygen reservoir, and not have a pop-off valve. A child bag has a reservoir of 450 ml, whereas an adult bag has a reservoir of at least 1000 ml.

[2] A neonatal mask is necessary for rescue units that may deliver a premature infant in the field.

[3] Many types of cervical immobilization devices are currently available, including wedges, collars, and so forth. The type of device used depends on local preference and policies and procedures. Whatever device is chosen should be stocked in a variety of sizes to fit infants, children, adolescents, and adults. The use of sandbags to meet this requirement is discouraged, because they may cause injury if a patient has to be turned.

[4] A thermal blanket may help to minimize heat loss. Hypothermia will complicate many illnesses and injuries, particularly in infants and young children. The type of material used depends on local preference, protocols, and procedures but may include Mylar, standard blankets, or aluminum foil for small infants.

[5] Infants should be restrained in ambulances. Car seats may be used for medical emergencies or in trauma when the infant is already restrained in a seat and not critically injured. Traumatically injured infants should be restrained on a gurney if they are not already in a seat. Many types of seats are available to meet this guideline. A recently developed seat that is collapsible and easy to store. The type of seat that is procured will be determined by local preference, policy, and procedure.

[6] A nasopharyngeal airway may be useful when the upper airway compromises respiration and an oral airway cannot be secured. Physicians must be trained in its use and know the contraindications for insertion of this device.

Table 17.

ALS Ambulance Pediatric Supplies and Equipment

All ALS ambulances should carry everything on the BLS list in Table 16 plus the following equipment and supplies:

Essential

Transport monitor
Defibrillator with adult and pediatric paddles[1]
Monitoring electrodes, pediatric sizes
Laryngoscope with straight blades, sizes 0–2, and curved blades, sizes 2–4
Pediatric- and adult-size endotracheal tube stylets
Endotracheal tubes: uncuffed sizes, 2.5–6.0; cuffed sizes, 6.0–8.0
Magill forceps, pediatric and adult
Nasogastric tubes, 8F–16F[2]
Nebulizer
Intravenous catheters, 16–24 g
Intraosseous needles
Length- and weight-based drug dose chart or tape[3]
Needles, 20–25 g
Resuscitation drugs and intravenous fluids that meet the local standard of practice

Desirable

Blood-glucose analysis system[4]
CO_2 detection device (disposable)

[1] A defibrillator should be able to deliver from 5 to 360 joules. The addition of pediatric paddles may give the responding unit enhanced capabilities but is not essential for units that rarely use this equipment. The defibrillator may be equipped with only adult paddles/pads or pediatric paddles and adult paddles/pads. Units carrying only adult paddles/pads should ensure that physicians are trained in the proper use of adult paddles for infants and children. When the defibrillator cannot deliver a low dose of joules for infants, shock at the lowest possible energy level.

[2] Nasogastric tubes may be useful when the transport time is greater than 30 minutes for patients who have abdominal distention that may impede respiration.

[3] One example of a commercially available item that correlates length with weight to generate accurate drug doses and equipment needed for resuscitation is the Broselow tape. Other length and weight tapes or charts may be substituted for this device.

[4] Many EMS systems estimate blood glucose in the field. The accuracy of any single blood-glucose test is affected by many factors such as the shelf life of the particular strip used, how the blood sample was obtained, and the education of the physician using the skill. Quality improvement is an important component of any laboratory analysis and should be applied to this field procedure. Universal precautions must always be followed when handling blood.

what point in the delivery of care the provider is expected to contact medical direction. In contrast, standing orders are care directives that have been preauthorized by the medical director and do not require contact with medical direction before initiating treatment. An action such as defibrillating an adult in cardiac arrest with no pulse or giving oxygen to a child in respiratory distress are examples of standing orders. Nevertheless, the administration of specific medications in either of these cases may require contact with medical direction, depending on the protocol being used. Benefits of such a system are: education of EMS personnel regarding protocol selection or deviation, directed patient assessment, enhanced communication, and concurrent quality improvement.

Ideally both types of medical direction should be incorporated into the EMS system, but the size of the community, the number of interested physicians, the number of providers and ambulance responses, and state regulations, among other factors, determine which type of system is best for the locale.

Transport and Triage Decisions

When an ambulance has arrived at the scene and the providers have assessed the patient, provided initial care, and determined that transport to a hospital is appropriate, the decision about the appropriate receiving hospital is based on several factors.

Specialized centers such as pediatric and general trauma and burn centers, designated by state or regional requirements or legislation, have been in existence for several years. These centers have demonstrated improved outcomes in caring for such patients and can provide the EMS system with predetermined categories of patients who require transport to such hospitals instead of others that may be closer. Criteria to bypass another hospital in favor of a trauma center may be based on the presence of the following indications: abnormal vitals signs; evidence of shock or respiratory compromise; significant head trauma (Glasgow Coma Scale < 8); specific injuries sustained such as penetrating injury; to the head, neck or chest; evidence of spinal cord injury, limb-threatening injuries such as amputations; or high-energy mechanism of injury (motor vehicle crash with a speed > 35 mph, fall > 20 feet). Although there may be pediatric or children's hospitals in the region, the bypass categories for children tend to be system dependent. Regionalization and categorization systems of hospitals for pediatric patients, such as the designation of Emergency Departments Approved for Children (EDAP) and Pediatric Critical Care Centers (PCCC) as in Los Angeles, California, direct pediatric patients to the hospitals that have the appropriate personnel, training, equipment, supplies, medications, and support personnel needed to stabilize, and, in the case of a PCCC, treat a critically ill or injured child (see Chapter 10). The Los Angeles county EMS Agency developed this system and uses it to direct pediatric patients to the most appropriate facility and to bypass those that have not received such a designation.

How EMS-C Fits Into EMS and Where the Pediatrician Fits In

One of the goals of EMS-C is to integrate into the existing EMS system, not to create a parallel system. Whereas some of the steps may be in compliance with legislation on a federal, state, regional, or local level, the actual groundwork is done by those at the grassroots level. The participation of parents, the public, schools, healthcare physicians of all levels (out-of-hospital care providers, nurses, and physicians), EMS agencies, and hospitals (community, pediatric, and rehabilitation) in the EMS-C continuum of care can help integrate pediatric-specific goals into the EMS system.

Pediatric input into the development of the new NHTSA curriculum for EMT-Bs and EMT-Ps has resulted in increased emphasis on pediatric topics in the new curricula. However, the education of out-of-hospital care providers in pediatrics does not stop with their initial training. A list of topics and skills essential for pediatric education of paramedics has recently been developed (see Tables 18 and 19). This training can be accomplished, with the help of the pediatrician, through didactic training at the local EMS agency, ambulance base, or fire department and by developing office internships or clinical time for physicians through which they can gain pediatric assessment skills, learn more about normal childhood development, and receive anticipatory guidance for injury prevention.

Table 18.

Topics Essential for Pediatric Education of Paramedics
••

Patient assessment
Growth and development
Emergency Medical Services for Children (EMS-C)
Illness and injury prevention
Respiratory emergencies (airway and breathing problems)
   Respiratory distress, respiratory failure, respiratory arrest
   Possible causes
   Airway obstruction (upper and lower)
   Fluid in the lungs
Cardiovascular and circulatory emergencies
   Shock (compensated and uncompensated)
   Rate and rhythm disturbances, cardiopulmonary arrest
Altered mental status
   Possible causes
   Airway or breathing problems or both, shock, seizures, poisoning,
     metabolic causes, occult trauma, serious infection
Trauma
   Burns
Child abuse and neglect
Behavioral emergencies
   Suicide, aggressive behavior
Child-family communications
Critical incident stress management
Fever
Medicolegal issues
   DNR (do not resuscitate) orders, consent, guardianship, refusal of care
Newborn emergencies
Near-drowning
Pain management
Poisoning
SIDS (sudden infant death syndrome) and death in the field
Transport considerations
   Destination issues, methods for transport (safety seats and
     parental transport)
Infants and children with special needs
   Technology-assisted children (TAC)
   Apnea monitors, central lines, chronic illness, gastrostomy tubes,
     home artificial ventilators and shunts

••

Table 19.

Essential Skills for Pediatric Education of Paramedics

Assessment of infants and children
Use of a length-based resuscitation tape
Airway management
  Mouth-to-mouth barrier devices
  Oropharyngeal airway
  Nasopharyngeal airway
  Oxygen delivery system
  Bag-valve-mask ventilation
  Endotracheal intubation
  Optional: endotracheal placement confirmation devices (CO_2
      detection);
      rapid sequence induction
  Foreign-body removal with Magill forceps
  Needle thoracostomy
  Nasogastric or orogastric tubes
  Suctioning
  Tracheostomy management
Monitoring
  Cardiorespiratory monitoring
  Pulse oximetry
  End-tidal CO_2, monitoring or CO_2 detection or both
Vascular access
  Intravenous line placement
  Intraosseous line placement
Fluid and medication administration
  Endotracheal
  Intramuscular
  Intravenous
  Nasogastric
  Nebulized
  Oral
  Rectal
  Subcutaneous
Cardioversion
Defibrillation
Drug dosing in infants and children
Immobilization and extrication
  Car-seat extrication
  Spinal immobilization

Participate in medical direction by offering to examine pediatric-sized equipment and supplies that are available in the ambulance, and review the pediatric-specific protocols or standing orders. If none exist, offer to work with the EMS medical director to develop them, and use prior EMS-C products to assist you. If there is no medical direction for a BLS unit, offer assistance where you can (check state laws, inasmuch as some require an EMS medical director to be board certified in emergency medicine, whereas others require a licensed physician). Ask questions about where your patients are transported, and who makes these decisions. If there are specialized hospitals in your region, what bypass protocols exist (if any)? Does a pediatric emergency department or hospital categorization system exist in your area? Although it may not be practical in rural areas to implement such designation criteria, knowledge about their existence in other regions can provide you with examples of how to improve your local EMS system capabilities.

Take a field trip to the hospital's emergency department and talk to the emergency department director about its preparedness for pediatric emergencies. How does it compare with published guidelines? Ask what you can do to help. Offer to act as a pediatric consultant for the emergency department physicians (if you do not already provide this service for your patients). What transfer guidelines or criteria are in place, where do the patients go, which type of system (air or ground) is used, are specialized teams available (if so, what is their composition), and what arrangements are made for family members to reach the receiving hospital?

Summary

Whether a committee or a single person becomes the lightning rod to accomplish the tasks addressed in this chapter, the keys are knowledge of the existing EMS system, expertise in pediatrics, some time and energy, and a desire to have a system of optimal out-of-hospital care and EMS equipped to care for one's patients, children, neighbors, and community.

Suggested Reading

American Academy of Pediatrics Committee on Pediatric Emergency Medicine. Guidelines for pediatric emergency care facilities. *Pediatrics.* 1995;96:526–537

American College of Emergency Physicians. Minimum pediatric prehospital equipment guidelines. *ACEP News.* 1992;11:

American College of Emergency Physicians. Preparedness of the emergency department for the care of children. Policy statement. American College of Emergency Physicians, Dallas, TX, October 1993. Reaffirmed October 1997

Committee on Pediatric Emergency Medical Services, Institute of Medicine. *Emergency Medical Services for Children.* Washington, DC: National Academy Press; 1993

Delbridge TR, Verdile VP, Sullivan MP. Contemporary medical direction. In: Paris PM, Roth RN, Verdile VP, eds. *Prehospital Medicine: The Art of On-Line Medical Command.* St. Louis, MO: Mosby Year-Book; 1996:3–12

Gausche M, Henderson DP, Brownstein D, Foltin GL. The education of out-of-hospital emergency medical personnel in pediatrics: report of a national task force. *Prehosp Emerg Care.* 1998;2:56–61

Illinois Emergency Medical Services for Children. *Pediatric Resource Manual.* Chicago, IL: Illinois Department of Health; 1997

Kuehl A, ed. *Prehospital Systems and Medical Oversight.* 2nd ed. St. Louis, MO: C. V. Mosby Company; 1994

Martensen RL. The evolution of the modern ambulance. *JAMA.* 1997;277:273

National Emergency Medical Services for Children Resource Alliance Committee on Pediatric Equipment and Supplies for Emergency Departments. Guidelines for pediatric equipment and supplies for emergency departments. *Ann Emerg Med.* 1998;31:54–57

National Highway Traffic Safety Administration. *Emergency Medical Services: Agenda for the Future.* Washington, DC: National Highway Traffic Safety Administration; 1996

State of California Health and Welfare Agency. Emergency Medical Services Authority. Administration, personnel and policy guidelines for the care of pediatric patients in the emergency department. Sacramento, CA: California EMS Authority; February, 1994

State of California Health and Welfare Agency. Emergency Medical Services Authority. Interfacility pediatric trauma and critical care consultation and/or Transfer Guidelines. Sacramento, CA: California EMS Authority; February, 1994

State of California Health and Welfare Agency. Emergency Medical Services Authority. Prehospital pediatric equipment for BLS/ALS support units. Sacramento, CA: California EMS Authority; February, 1994

Stoy WA, Center for Emergency Medicine. *Mosby's EMT-Basic Textbook.* St. Louis, MO: Mosby Lifeline; 1996

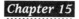

Children With Special Healthcare Needs and EMS-C

Key Points Concerning CSHCN

1. Eighteen percent of US children have special healthcare needs.

2. Children with special healthcare needs should have an emergency information form.

3. A comprehensive transitional-care plan helps the child return to home, school, and community with minimal problems.

Introduction

Advances in technology and care have improved survival for children with severe or complex medical problems. As a result, there is a growing population of children worldwide with special healthcare needs (CSHCN).

Emergency care, urgent care, and posthospital discharge transitional care for CSHCN are part of EMS-C. This chapter presents the definition of CSHCN, the use of the Emergency Information Form (EIF), the formulation of transitional-care plan, and other important EMS-C concerns in caring for CSHCN.

Definition of a Child With Special Healthcare Needs

The Maternal Child Health Bureau's Division of Services for Children with Special Health Care Needs Work Group defines CSHCN as follows:

CSHCN are those who have or are at increased risk for a chronic physical, developmental, behavioral, or emotional condition and who also require health and related services of a type or amount beyond that required by children generally.

Who Are the CSHCN?

A 1994 survey indicates that 12% of US children less than 18 years old have a chronic physical, developmental, behavioral, or emotional condition and need health or related services beyond those required by children generally. An additional 6% of children have a presumed need for health or related services beyond those required by the normal population. When the two groups, those with increased service use and those with presumed increased service needs, are combined, an estimated 18% of US children less than 18 years, or 12.6 million children nationally, have healthcare needs beyond those usually required by children.

The prevalence of CSHCN varies in relation to demographic and socioeconomic characteristics of the population. Prevalence increases in a step-by-step manner with age; school-aged children are twice as likely as toddlers to be classified as having an existing special need. Boys are about one-third more likely than girls to have a special need. Differences are also apparent in relation to race and ethnicity. African American children are most likely and Hispanic children are less likely than white children to be categorized as having an existing special need.

Children from families with incomes at or below the federal poverty level ($12 320 for a family of three in 1994) are about one-third more likely than children from families above the federal poverty level to have an existing special healthcare need. Educational level of the head of the household also correlates with the presence of a special-health-needs child, with a higher prevalence in lower socioeconomic groups. Children in single parent families are about 40% more likely than children from two-parent households to have existing special healthcare needs.

Thirty-one percent of children experience chronic conditions of a physical nature. Nearly 7% of children experience limitations in social-role activities, such as school or play, because of chronic physical or mental conditions. A much smaller proportion of children, 0.2% nationwide, need assistance or special equipment for performing the activities of daily living (eating, bathing, dressing, etc.). About 1 in every 1000 children is institutionalized because of chronic health problems.

Health Characteristics of CSHCN

There are substantial differences between children with and without special healthcare needs with regard to health status, access to care, and use of health services (Table 20). CSHCN spend three times as many days ill in bed and are absent from school three times as many days as other children. These differences in rates translate into 52 million days spent ill in bed and 58 million days of absence from school annually.

Table 20.

Children With Special Healthcare Needs Compared With All Children and With Children Without Special Healthcare Needs by Categories of Health Status, Access to Care, and Use of Health Services: United States, 1994

	All Children	Children With Special Healthcare Needs	Children Without Special Healthcare Needs
Health Status			
Average annual bed days due to illness	2.8	6.1	2.0
Average annual school absences due to illness	3.6	7.4	2.8
Access to Care			
Percentage with health insurance	86.8	88.8	86.4
Percentage with a usual source of care	93.4	94.4	93.2
Percentage not satisfied with their usual source of care	14.7	17.9	13.6
Percentage with one or more unmet health needs	7.6	12.9	6.4
Use of Health Services			
Average annual physician contacts	3.3	6.4	2.6
Percentage hospitalized in past year	3.1	7.4	2.2
Average annual hospital days per 1000 children	225.0	691.0	122.0

An estimated 11.2% of CSHCN are uninsured. More than 5% do not have a source of primary care. Nearly 20% of parents report dissatisfaction with at least one dimension of care provided to their children with existing special healthcare needs. In general, rates of parental dissatisfaction with care are higher for CSHCN than for other children.

CSHCN have more than twice as many physician contacts and five times as many hospital bed days as do other children.

Emergency Information Form (EIF)

Specialty and primary-care physicians may not be available for immediate consultation with physicians providing emergency care for their patients with special healthcare needs. To improve care for CSHCN, the American College of Emergency Physicians (ACEP) and the American Academy of Pediatrics (AAP) recommend utilization of the Emergency Information Form. The EIF is intended to be a concise, readily available information source that provides a summary of the child's medical history, physical findings, and important and unique management requirements. It is completed by the patient's specialist, pediatrician, or family-care physician. For a patient who has several physicians providing specialty care, a single specialist or the child's primary-care physician should be responsible for completion and revision of the EIF.

An example of a completed EIF is illustrated in Figure 23. The elements of the EIF are:

- *Introductory information, medical history, and current health status.* This section of the form contains basic demographic information, identifies the child's physicians, and provides their telephone numbers. It also contains a space for noting the latest revisions in the patient's plan of care.
- *Child's medical history.* This section concisely describes the aspects of the child's anatomy and physiology that are important in the provision of emergency care.

- *Diagnosis.* This section lists the medical diagnoses. All abbreviations should be defined.
- *Synopsis.* A brief description of the patient's current problems are presented in this section. The description is intended to be educational and to note conditions unique to the patient. Relevant history may be included in this section but only as it applies to the child's immediate conditions. Include past problems that may recur, but exclude information with little relevance to emergency care.
- *Significant baseline physical and ancillary findings.* These sections are used to list those findings normal for this child that would be abnormal in other children; for example, central cyanosis in a child with congenital heart disease.
- *Management data.* This section provides information on immediate care of the child. The purpose of this section is to facilitate immediate and appropriate treatment of the special-needs child in the emergency department.
- *Medications and procedures to be avoided and why.* List any medications or procedures that may be dangerous for this particular child, as well as a very brief explanation of why the medication or procedure should not be used.
- *Antibiotic prophylaxis.* This section should include the indications and doses of antibiotics.
- *Common presenting problems and suggested management.* The last section of the EIF is provided for the specialist to list common presenting problems that require special consideration. Include diagnostic studies or management techniques that are not normally used in children presenting with similar complaints. This section is also used to note those physical or ancillary findings that are not normally present in this child but signify a major problem and tests that may not be necessary to obtain for emergency care.
- *Comments.* Any general instructions unique to this particular patient or the child's family or social situation may be included in this section.

Emergency Information Form for Children With Special Needs

▦ American College of Emergency Physicians®	American Academy of Pediatrics ⚫	Date form 1/1/97 completed By Whom J. Heart, MD	Revised 5/15/98 Initials JH Revised Initials

---

Name: Blue, Little B.   Birth date: 7/4/96   Nickname: LB

Home Address: 1313 Mockingbird Lane, Anytown, USA, 11111   Home/Work Phone: 900-555-1212 (home) 777-8899 (work)

Parent/Guardian: Sandra Blue, mother   Emergency Contact Names & Relationship: Beatrice Blue,

Signature/Consent*: *Sandra Blue*   grandmother

Primary Language: English   Phone Number(s): 900-444-5566

Physicians:

Primary care physician: Marcus Welby, MD   Emergency Phone: 1-800-KIDS-RUS

                                                  Fax: 000-000-0000

Current Specialty physician: P. Card. Jime Heart, MD   Emergency Phone: 000-000-0000
Specialty:
                                                  Fax: 000-000-0000

Current Specialty physician: P. Neuro. Joe Neuro, MD   Emergency Phone: 000-000-0000
Specialty:
                                                  Fax: 000-000-0000

Anticipated Primary ED: Smallville Hospital   Pharmacy:

Anticipated Tertiary Care Center: Childrens All Star Regional Med Center

---

Diagnoses/Past Procedures/Physical Exam:

1 . tetralogy of Fallot with pulmonary atresia; RV to PA   Baseline physical findings: gr III harsh murmur, few crackles

   conduit 2/97 VSD left, ductus and collaterals ligated   at base of left lung, liver down 5 cm.

2. Asplenia syndrome

3. thrombosed bilat femoral, iliac veins and inferior   Baseline vital signs: P 90 BP 100/50 R 24, O$_2$ Sat 85%

   vena cava   Weight: 12 kg   Date: 5/15/98

4. Seizure disorder: generalized tonic-clonic

Synopsis: Asymptomatic, mildly cyanotic nb. Asplenia

syndrome noted. Surgery of RV to PA conduit at   Baseline neurological status: Awake , age appropriate,

8 mos. of age. Post-op seizures-mild R CVA, hemiparesis   interactive. Mild increased tone L>R. EEG 5/97: Mild

resolved.   assymetry with right-sided slowing

*Consent for release of this form to health care providers

Fig 23. Example of completed EIF for CSHCN.

Diagnoses/Past Procedures/Physical Exam continued:

Medications:	Significant baseline ancillary findings (lab, x-ray, ECG):
1. Digoxin 50 mcg=1cc BID	moderate cardiomegaly on cxr
2. Lasix 10 mg BID	chronic LLL atelectasis on cxr
3. Amoxil 200 mg BID	RVH on EkG
4. Phenobarb 40 mg BID	Prostheses/Appliances/Advanced Technology Devices: homograft
5.	conduit RV to MPA — no extra precautions. Sternal wires
6.	and clips on vessels — no MRI until 6 mos post-op

Management Data:

Allergies: Medications/Foods to be avoided	and why:
1. Betadine	rash
2.	
3.	

Procedures to be avoided	and why:
1. femoral venous puncture	no fem veins
2. instillation of air into venous catheters	R to L intracardiac shunt
3.	

Immunizations

Dates	9/4/96	11/4/96	1/4/97	1/10/98		Dates	9/4/96	11/4/96	1/4/97	1/10/98	
DPT	X	X	X	X		Hep B		X			
OPV	X	X	X	X		Varicella					
MMR				X		TB status					
HIB	X	X	X			Other				Pneumovax	

Antibiotic prophylaxis: Indication: Asplenia   Medication and dose: Amoxil 200 mg BID
                          SBE Prophylaxis   Amoxil 50 mg/kg one hour prior to procedure

Common Presenting Problems/Findings With Specific Suggested Managements

Problem	Suggested Diagnostic Studies	Treatment Considerations
Worsened CHF	cxr	increase lasix
Status Epilepticus	check electrolytes-Na check phenobarbitol level	midazolam, correct lytes
Fever	sepsis w/u	broad spectrum atbx for asplenic individual

Comments on child, family, or specific medical issues: Mother is an excellent caregiver a nd knows when

LB is blue.

Physician/Provider Signature: *Jime Heart MD*   Print Name: Jime Heart, MD

The EIF must be available 24 hours a day, independent of the accessibility of the patient's specialist or designee. Emergency department retrieval, either by facsimile transmission or by computer interface, must be available through a continuously available server. Possible sources for such a service include existing medical information repositories such as the Medic Alert Foundation, regional Poison Control Centers, regional Emergency Medical Services Command Centers, dedicated EIF Centers, and after hours call centers. A 24-hour-staffed center with facsimile transmission capabilities provides the widest access to the EIF system. Even the most remote emergency department or physician's office can have facsimile transmission capabilities.

Encourage parents of CSHCN to provide some form of identification to notify healthcare physicians of their problems. This identification should be evident even if the patient is not accompanied by an adult or is unable to communicate. Medical jewelry has proved effective as an identifier and has been used very successfully by existing information services. Such identification jewelry should alert the healthcare physician that a problem exists and that an EIF is available through a specified telephone number.

The EIF is also designed to be an out-of-hospital tool, and systems should be established for out-of-hospital providers to access the EIF information in a timely fashion. For out-of-hospital use, the EIF can identify hospitals preferred for emergency care.

Recommendations for Coordination of Care for CSHCN

The EMS-C National Task Force on CSHCN makes recommendations that emphasize the need for coordination of care. A summary of the key recommendations follows.

- Identify the CSHCN early (Table 21). Identification will allow maximal time to prepare a complete transitional plan for care after discharge.
- Provide assistance for families of CSHCN in identifying sources of appropriate emergency and continuing care.
- Develop protocols for completing and updating the EIF.
- Coordinate follow-up care and services required for transition from hospital to school and community.

- Include physical medicine and rehabilitation professionals in each child's medical treatment. Encourage active participation in the child's care as soon as possible after initial stabilization.
- Contact the child's primary-care physician from the emergency department or early in a child's hospitalization, and provide details of the child's medical status.
- Include the primary-care physician in decision-making regarding the child's emergency and ongoing care. The primary-care physician, his or her designee, or a designated coordinator on the medical treatment team should have responsibility for ensuring that the details of the transitional-care plan are completed.
- Link any child or family without an established medical physician with a primary-care physician.

Table 21.

Guidelines for Identifying Which CSHCN Will Benefit From Transitional and Ongoing Care

Use the CSHCN definition to identify a child who has special healthcare needs and who meets one or more of the following criteria:

- Depends on medical technology, such as a ventilator, broviac catheter, or infusion pump. Has a preexisting condition that causes progressive changes in health status or functional abilities.
- Exhibits a neurologic, musculoskeletal, or developmental disability, including delayed development of age-appropriate functions requiring cognitive, motor, communicative, behavioral, social, or emotional skills.
- Requires medication, hospice care, home health care, rehabilitation therapy, or other specialized medical or therapeutic interventions.
- Has sustained a brain injury, spinal cord injury, submersion injury, burn, multiple fractures, physical disfigurement, or loss of a limb.
- Has a seizure disorder.
- Has injuries suggestive of abuse or neglect.
- Has been a victim or witness of violence.
- Experiences sudden, uncontrollable behavioral or emotional changes such as aggression or withdrawal.

Seamless Care for CSHCN: Developing the Transitional-Care Plan

A transitional plan anticipates the posthospital-discharge needs of CSHCN. Creating a transitional-care plan requires organization (Tables 21 through 23). Steps in the development of a transitional plan include:

1. *Identify members of the transitional-care team.* Family participation is the cornerstone of effective transitional care. The family must take an active role in all aspects of planning and decision-making.

   Early participation in patient care by rehabilitation professionals may help reduce the disabling effect of some conditions.

2. *Designate a care coordinator.* Designate one person as the primary-care coordinator, or case manager. The coordinator is responsible for overseeing and following through on the recommendations outlined in the transitional-care plan. The coordinator informs the family of available community resources and provides it with written information detailing the child's condition. It is important that this information be supplied in a form that the family can refer to easily.

   The coordinator's responsibilities include assisting with health-insurance benefits and helping the family find appropriate contacts in the medical and education systems. The AAP has published a policy on CSHCN and managed care. The coordinator should also promote communication between the child's family, primary-care physician, and school well before the child's discharge from the hospital.

3. *Formulate the transitional-care plan for the child's environment and family resources.* The primary-care physician and the medical treatment team must consider every environment where the child will spend time, including the home, the school, and recreational facilities. Make a plan for any special equipment or procedures that may be necessary for the safety and well-being of the child. The plan should also include provisions for individualized education and emergency care, a mechanism for evaluating family preparedness, and provisions for counseling and dispensing information about strategies to prevent injury or illness.

The transitional-care plan should take into consideration family training and education as well as any special skills that family members will need to care for the child.

4. *Prepare an emergency-care plan.* CSHCN require emergency and urgent care. Often, this care will be provided by a health-care physician who is unfamiliar with the patient's medical history. Caretakers are not always able to accurately relay vital information on the essential medical needs of the children in their care. This problem may be compounded in emergency situations. Have the team and family develop an emergency-care plan that specifies any actions to be taken in a crisis sit-uation and includes an updated medical record such as the EIF. All the CSHCN caretakers and others who take part in the child's daily activities should become familiar with the emer-gency-care plan. Have copies of the plan available wherever the child spends time.

Families of children with particular risks or ongoing health-care requirements need basic life-support training.

Send notification letters to local utility companies and emergency services to inform them of the child's special healthcare needs and what should be done in the event of an emergency. Specific groups and people who should know about this emergency-care plan include: 911 dispatchers, emergency medical services and fire departments, school nurses and administrators, and the child's physicians and therapists. Supply a copy of the EIF to the emergency depart-ment to which the child usually-goes for care.

Help families obtain an identification bracelet or necklace. The use of some form of independent identification and infor-mation set, such as the EIF, is needed to ensure proper treat-ment of CSHCN. The EIF is available through the AAP or ACEP. Other model emergency-care plans have been developed through grant programs funded through the federal EMS-C program (see Chapter 26).

Table 22.

Guidelines for Identifying the Types of Assistance That May Be Needed

• Help to obtain services and payment resources to meet the child's healthcare needs. A liaison with health, social, and educational services.
• Support services to help families adjust emotionally to the child's changing health status and the demands of providing appropriate care.
• Education related to home healthcare for the child.
• Teaching families and providing information about illness or injury prevention. Housing modifications to accommodate the child's new or chronic disability.

Table 23.

Essential Components in Creating Care Plans for CSHCN

Primary healthcare physician
Title V programs
Social services
Specialty health services
Rehabilitation services
Transitional care
Home healthcare
Home equipment
Protective resources
Psychological services
Schools
Vocational education and rehabilitation
Healthcare insurer
Financial assistance
Alternative resources

Summary

Transitional and emergency care of CSHCN are important components of the federal EMS-C program. Early identification and an organized approach facilitate transitional planning. Completion of the EIF aids emergency-care physicians regarding a child's special problems or needs. Additional information on CSHCN can be found in the EMS-C Five Year Plan and by contacting the National EMS-C Resource Center.

Suggested Reading

American Academy of Pediatrics Committee on Children with Disabilities. Managed care and children with special health care needs: a subject review. *Pediatrics.* 1998;102:657–660

American Academy of Pediatrics Committee on Children with Disabilities and Committee on Adolescence. Transition of care provided for adolescents with special health care needs. *Pediatrics.* 1996;98:1203–1206

Carraccio CL, Dettmer KS, duPont ML, et al. Family member knowledge of children's medical problems: the need for universal application of an emergency information form. *Pediatrics.* 1998;102:367–370

Emergency Medical Services for Children, National Task Force on Children with Special Health Care Needs. EMS for children: recommendations for coordinating care for children with special health care needs. *Ann Emerg Med.* 1997;30:274–280

Gunby P. Test of new medical dog tag with civilian potential. *JAMA.* 1998;279:99–100

McPherson M, Arango P, Fox H, et al. A new definition of children with special health care needs. *Pediatrics.* 1998;102:137–140

Newacheck PW, Strickland B, Shonkoff JP, et al. An epidemiologic profile of children with special health care needs. *Pediatrics.* 1998;102:117–123

Sacchetti A, Gerardi M, Barkin R, et al. Emergency information form for children with special needs. *Ann Emerg Med.* 1996;28:324–327

US Department of Health and Human Services, Health Resources and Services Administration, Maternal and Child Health Bureau, National Highway Traffic Safety Administration. *5 Year Plan: Midcourse Review— Emergency Medical Services for Children, 1995–2000.* Washington DC: Emergency Medical Services for Children National Resource Center; 1997

Chapter 16

Disasters, Mass Casualty Events, and Disaster Preparedness

Key Points in Planning for Disasters

1. Children must be included in disaster planning.

2. The Joint Commission on Accreditation of Healthcare Organizations requires hospitals to participate in mock disasters twice a year.

3. Pediatricians can educate parents in disaster preparation and planning.

4. Many state and national resources are available.

Introduction

Although dealing with disasters is not part of a pediatrician's daily routine, 1.5 million households in the United States experience injury or suffer property damage each year from natural disasters. Events such as an organophosphate exposure in Arizona, hurricanes Hugo, Iniki, and Andrew, the Loma Prieta and Northridge earthquakes, the Los Angeles riots, the Oklahoma City bombing, and tornadoes in Arkansas and Florida have provided a perspective on the needs of children and the challenges facing pediatricians in disasters and mass casualty events. The physical legacy of a disaster may be serious and widespread. The emotional effect may persist well after the physical signs are gone. The focus of this chapter is to help the primary physician better prepare to assess and treat children and families in the event of a disaster.

Basic Disaster Nomenclature and Response

A *disaster* is an event that destroys property, includes injury or loss of life, and affects a large population or area. Disasters are usually described as (1) natural, including earthquakes, hurricanes, tornadoes, and floods; and (2) manmade, including fire, mass-transportation incidents, environmental toxins, and civil unrest. More narrowly defined and distinct is a *mass casualty incident* (MCI), an event that causes a large number of injuries but does not threaten or harm large segments of the community.

Each disaster differs in its effects. Considerations are given to the *size of the area* affected, the *extent of the damage,* and the *effect on community resources.* The extent of damage includes the physical injury and damage to property, especially destruction of infrastructure (roadways, bridges, telephones). The effects on community resources include (1) absence of electricity, gas, sanitation, and potable water and (2) potential for recurrence (eg, earthquakes with aftershocks or ongoing damage from floods or hurricanes). Other effects on the community may include loss of community cohesion, increased vulnerability, exploitation due to the disaster, and media sensationalism.

The planning for and response to disasters traditionally falls to federal, state, and local governments. The Federal Emergency Management Agency (FEMA) responds to declared national emergencies, providing Disaster Medical Assistant Teams (DMATs). DMATs are locally based volunteer organizations that are equipped and trained, under local sponsorship with federal coordination. DMATs are deployed to disaster sites with sufficient supplies and equipment to sustain themselves for a period of 72 hours while providing medical care at a fixed or medical-care site. DMATs may provide primary healthcare or may serve to augment overloaded local healthcare staffs or both. A DMAT is made up of professional and paraprofessional medical personnel and is designed to be a rapid-response element to supplement local medical care until other resources can be mobilized or the situation is resolved. DMAT members are required to maintain appropriate certification and licensing. When activated, they are protected under the Federal Tort Claims Act. Professionals interested in joining a DMAT may contact the National Disaster Medical System headquarters at (800) 872-6367. Information on starting a DMAT may be requested at the same number.

Other federal agencies dealing with disaster preparedness and management include the Department of Transportation, the Department of Defense, the Department of Housing and Urban Development, the Department of Agriculture, and the Federal Aviation Administration (Table 24). On a regional level, state and local emergency management authorities (often within the state or local department of health services) have areawide response plans. These authorities organize emergency operation centers

(EOCs) whose duties include: (1) hospital damage assessment; (2) allocation, designation, and distribution of casualty collection points (CCPs); (3) identification, prevention, and elimination of public health hazards; (4) coordination of activities with support departments and public utilities; and, (5) coordination of requests for mutual aid. (For a list of State Emergency Management directors, see Appendix 4 at the end of this chapter or contact the FEMA Web site.)

Hospitals are required by the Joint Commission on Accreditation of Healthcare Organizations (JCAHO) to have a disaster plan in place and to practice the plan twice a year. These plans include the hospital's response to mass casualty incidents and to internal disasters such as fire, loss of utilities, and so forth. The responsibilities of physicians and other professionals are usually included under the hospital disaster plan.

Volunteer organizations such as the Red Cross and the Salvation Army have key roles in disaster response. The services provided by these organizations include disaster planning, disaster preparedness, community disaster education, mitigation, and

Table 24.

Primary Functions of Lead Federal Agencies in Disaster Management

Function	Lead Agency
Transportation	Department of Transportation
Communications	National Communication Agency
Public works/engineering	US Army Corps of Engineers
Fire fighting	Department of Agriculture
Planning/information	Federal Emergency Management Agency
Mass care	American Red Cross
Resource support	General Services Administration
Health and medical services	Department of Health and Human Services
Urban search and rescue	Federal Emergency Management Agency
Hazardous materials	Environmental Protection Agency
Food	Department of Agriculture
Energy	Department of Energy

response. The Red Cross provides shelter and food, individual and family assistance, and health and mental health services; it also contacts family members within the disaster area. In addition, recent recommendations include planning for disasters at the neighborhood, family, and personal level.

Children in a disaster environment may suffer a sense of loss (home, family, friends, pets, and possessions), sustain physical injury, and develop acute or chronic stress-induced problems. An understanding of children and family dynamics is needed to deal appropriately with disasters. Information on the psychosocial problems can be found in the AAP Work Group on Disasters document titled "Psychosocial Issues for Children and Families in Disasters: A Guide for the Primary Care Physician." The pediatrician can provide the expertise to address the needs and special problems of children in all three phases of a disaster: (1) before, (2) during and immediately after (day 0–2), and (3) during the aftermath and recovery (from day 3 on).

Planning Before a Disaster

A pediatrician should participate in community disaster plan development at all levels. AAP chapters should contribute information to the state and local offices of EMS to ensure that the needs of children are incorporated into every plan. The pediatrician should take part in local community response team planning to identify the numerous problems that disasters pose. Responses to drills and experiences from previous potentially similar disasters can be applied to preparation for future events. Assisting a community in preparing for a disaster may include providing anticipatory guidance to parents in the course of regular health visits and to schoolteachers in formal presentations. Such guidance may include the location of local shelters, reviewing first-aid tips, and reviewing symptoms that may arise in a child or adolescent after a disaster. Help determine and arrange for the necessary equipment for children to be available in shelters, ambulances, and emergency departments.

Lessons learned from recent disasters emphasize that fire, police, and other response agencies may be overburdened. Neighborhood groups may have to take initial emergency response actions and fend for themselves for 72 hours or longer.

Training programs for community response teams in basic emergency response techniques have been developed in several areas of California to prepare for loss of community services (see Appendix 1 at the end of this chapter). Although community physicians often volunteer after disasters, the response is often neither organized nor coordinated through official disaster agencies. If response is unorganized and uncoordinated, questions of liability also must be considered. The pediatrician should have an ongoing role in the EMS system by (1) training first responders in pediatric assessment, (2) assisting in the development of out-of-hospital pediatric protocols, (3) helping to establish protocols for minor's consent and identification, and (4) ensuring the availability of pediatric equipment.

Pediatric staff in local or regional children's hospitals may already be taking part in the development of the disaster plan. However, such participation may not be the case for general hospitals. It is important that local pediatricians meet with hospital staff members responsible for implementing the hospital disaster plan, review the plan, and learn the roles of the team members. Make sure that the plan addresses the needs of children and their families. The plan should incorporate pediatric resources such as emergency departments, burn units, trauma centers, and intensive care units. It should contain components for notification of parents, possible transfer to other special resource facilities, and procedures for discharge. Other components of the plan should include:

1. Specific guidelines for activation of the plan. These guidelines include information about who will have the authority to activate the plan, under what circumstances it should be activated, and how the hospital will implement the plan.
2. Provisions for the effective use of space, the procurement of additional supplies, the establishment of efficient communication between areas of the hospital, and increased security.
3. Provisions for the management of staff, including distribution and assignment of responsibilities and functions. Specific notification of additional or key personnel and shift and off-time management.
4. Provisions for movement of existing emergency-department and hospitalized patients who are not disaster victims (ie,

early discharge and arrangements for return follow-up at the hospital or by the primary-care physician).

5. Provisions for the management of patients, including triage, scheduling of services, control of patient information, notification of parents, admission, transfer, and discharge. Pediatric patients require larger staffs, as well as space for extended family members.

6. Provisions for the management of deceased patients.

7. Training of the staff on the details of the plan and their roles during emergencies.

8. A method to periodically test the plan that includes a written evaluation.

Community pediatricians can be used to both triage and treat patients during disasters. Important questions to ask include: (1) Where should the pediatrician go during the disaster? (2) How should pediatricians be notified (disaster trees, check in) when they are to perform their roles? (3) How should hospital physicians who will go to the scene be identified and notified? (4) How should pediatric transfers and discharges be handled? In addition, consider alternatives to the loss of power and conventional telephones. Back-up systems such as cellular telephones, direct lines that are not part of the regular telephone system, two-way radios, beepers, and citizens band radios should be considered. In areas where pediatricians cover several hospitals, initiate pools through the county medical or pediatric society to provide uniform pediatric coverage of area hospitals.

The pediatrician can aid schools and child care centers in developing disaster plans. Some states have laws that require that state-licensed child care facilities and schools develop and maintain a disaster and mass casualty plan. The University of Illinois at Urbana-Champaign has developed school activities for children before and after disaster. This resource guide includes activities, a curriculum on disasters and disaster preparedness, and a bibliography of children's literature on natural disasters. The Web site includes other helpful links (see Appendixes 1 and 3 at the end of this chapter).

In many areas, the office or clinic may become a site for care if area hospitals are out of service. Recent experiences have demonstrated how after-disaster healthcare may be administered in parking lots, malls, and tents, with limited power and water sources. Local offices may be unusable and alternative sites for primary care have to be identified. Prepare, regularly update, and practice an office disaster plan addressing response and recovery. Make office training programs in emergency procedures including first aid, cardiopulmonary resuscitation (CPR), evacuation, search and rescue, and the use of fire extinguishers a routine occurrence. It may be advisable to consult local building codes to ensure that the pediatrician's office building meets current structural safety standards. Obtain agreements with vendors for postdisaster operations. Assemble emergency kits with water, first-aid supplies, radios, flashlights, batteries, heavy gloves, food, and sanitation supplies.

In many areas of the United States, there is an ongoing threat of natural disasters. In these areas, anticipatory guidance on home disaster preparedness can be provided in the pediatric office or as a community focus. Family preparedness includes: CPR training, rendezvous points, lists of emergency telephone numbers, and an out-of-state friend or relative whom all family members can call after the event to report whereabouts and conditions. Home preparedness such as storm windows or earthquake proofing should be covered. Parents should maintain supplies of emergency food, water, and other essentials, including medicine, a first-aid kit, and clothing. Patients and their families should know the safest place in the house or apartment complex, make any special provisions, know community resources, and have a plan to reunite. Children with developmental disabilities or physical handicaps and those on medications for chronic illness may need added care, owing to the interruption of their routine care, the loss of facilities (such as handicap-access buildings), or the worsening of their conditions secondary to the disaster. These children and families should be targeted for predisaster planning, as well as outreach after the disaster, to ensure that facilities and equipment will be available (see Appendix 2 at the end of this chapter).

Action During a Disaster

The pediatrician's role during a disaster is determined by the disaster plan. Familiarity with the plan is paramount. Once the disaster is recognized, first institute office and home disaster plans, and then participate in the community or hospital plan as a scene, hospital, or clinic resource. The pediatrician may take part in disaster triage, direct patient care (including adults), patient discharge or transfer or both, facilitation and reception of patients at other sites including offices, and hospital evacuation. Studies from several recent disasters reveal that the number of patients in the emergency departments of affected hospitals increased by 15% to 40%. Minor trauma was the most common diagnosis, with an increased need in physician staffing because of wound management. Hospitalization may remain normal or increase only slightly, depending on the disaster.

Helping in the Aftermath of a Disaster

The period of recovery may be short or quite prolonged, depending on the nature of the disaster. Be prepared to deal with continued disruption of services, which will affect your ability to care for patients. Have plans to provide on-site emergency and primary healthcare to children in shelters. Problems to be addressed include inpatient and outpatient treatment, infectious disease control, alternatives for lost services and utilities, logistics and resupply, physical rehabilitation, mental rehabilitation, and critical-incident-stress debriefing. The primary-care physician in the community may also be coping with personal losses and problems. This role conflict poses a double burden and should not be ignored. The need to treat more patients with fewer supplies in a less than optimal treatment setting may take its toll on all caregivers. If the physician's office is damaged or destroyed in the disaster, rebuilding the structure and practice is a necessity. In the aftermath, changes in practice location, a lack of refrigeration for medications and vaccinations, continued disruption of communications, power outages, lack of sanitation, and so forth will force changes in practice standards and require inventiveness and flexibility. Assisting families in coping with the emotional toll of the disaster may be an ongoing responsibility of the pediatrician. The possible effects of a disaster on the family include death or physical injury to family members, loss of the family dwelling or possessions, relocation, job loss, and parental disorganization or dysfunction. The pediatrician must keep in mind that children and families are having a normal reaction to an abnormal situation. From a practical standpoint, with the closing of schools postdisaster, caregivers may need additional child care. Temporary housing also may be necessary for those healthcare workers who remain and help to rebuild the community.

Summary

The following lists summarize what a physician caring for children should do in the event of a disaster.

Before a Disaster

- Take part in community response planning.
- Prepare for loss of community services.
- Assist in the development of out-of-hospital pediatric protocols.
- Ensure availability of pediatric resources.
- Assist in the development or revision of hospital disaster plans.
- Aid in the development of school and child care plans.
- Prepare an office disaster plan.
- Provide anticipatory guidance.

During a Disaster

- Institute office and home disaster plans.
- Participate in community or hospital plan.

Aftermath Period and Recovery

- Prepare for continued disruption of services.
- Provide emergency and primary healthcare at emergency shelters.
- Provide physical and mental rehabilitation.
- Address as-needed inpatient and outpatient services, lost services and utilities, and logistics and resupply.

Suggested Reading

Aghababian R, Lewis CP, Gans L, Curley FJ. Disasters within hospitals. *Ann Emerg Med.* 1994;23:771–777

Alson RL, Leonard RB, Stringer LW. Disaster response in North Carolina. *N C Med J.* 1997;58:248–252

American Academy of Pediatrics Committee on Pediatric Emergency Medicine. The pediatrician's role in disaster preparedness. *Pediatrics.* 1997;99:130–133

American Academy of Pediatrics Committee on Psychosocial Aspects of Child and Family Health. How pediatricians can respond to the psychosocial implications of disasters. *Pediatrics.* 1999;103:521–523.

American Academy of Pediatrics Work Group on Disasters. *Psychosocial Issues for Children and Families in Disasters: A Guide for the Primary Care Physician.* Washington, DC: U.S. Department of Health and Human Services, Public Health Service, Substance Abuse and Mental Health Services Administration, Center for Mental Health Services; 1995

Auf der Heide E. Disaster planning, II: disaster problems, issues, and challenges identified in the research literature. *Emerg Med Clin North Am.* 1996;14:453–480

Auf der Heide E. *Disaster Response Principles of Preparation and Coordination.* St. Louis, MO: Mosby; 1989

Bissell RA, Becker BM, Burkle FM. Health care personnel in disaster response: reversible roles or territorial imperative? *Emerg Med Clin North Am.* 1996;14:267–288

Burkle FM. Triage. In: *Disaster Medicine,* (Burkle FM, Sanner PH, Wolcott BW, eds.) Medical Examination Publishing Co, Inc; New Hyde Park, NY: 1984:45-80

Conover WA. Earthquakes and the office-based surgeon. *West J Med.* 1992;157:79–82

Haynes BE, Freeman C, Rubin JL, Koehler GA, Enriquez SM, Smiley DR. Medical response to catastrophic events: California's planning and the Loma Prieta earthquake. *Ann Emerg Med.* 1992;21:368–374

Henderson AK, Lillibridge SR, Salinas C, Graves RW, Roth PB, Noji EK. Disaster medical assistance teams: providing health care to a community struck by hurricane Iniki. *Ann Emerg Med.* 1994;23:726–730

Howard MJ, Brillman JC, Burkle FM Jr. Infectious disease emergencies in disasters. *Emerg Med Clin North Am.* 1996;14:413–428

Leonard RB. Role of pediatricians in disasters and mass casualty incidents. *Ped Emerg Care.* 1988;4:41–44

Lewis CP, Aghababian RV. Disaster planning, I: overview of hospital and emergency department planning for internal and external disasters. *Emerg Med Clin North Am.* 1996;14:439–452

Noji EK. Disaster epidemiology. *Emerg Med Clin North Am.* 1996; 14:289–300

Noji EK. The medical consequences of earthquakes: coordinating the medical and rescue response. *Disaster Management.* 1991;4:32–40

Pointer JE, Michaelis J, Saunders C, et al. The 1989 Loma Prieta earthquake: impact on hospital care. *Ann Emerg Med.* 1992;21:1228–1233

Pretto EA Jr, Safar P. National medical response to mass disasters in the United States: are we prepared? *JAMA.* 1991;266:1259–1262

Quinn B, Baker R, Pratt J. Hurricane Andrew and a pediatric emergency department. *Ann Emerg Med.* 1994;23:737–741

Reitherman R. How to prepare a hospital for an earthquake. *J Emerg Med.* 1986;4:119–131

Roth PB. Status of a national disaster medical response. *JAMA.* 1991;266:1266

Roth PB, Gaffney JK. The federal response plan and disaster medical assistance teams in domestic disasters. *Emerg Med Clin North Am.* 1996;14:371–382

Roth PB, Vogel A, Key G, Hall G, Stockhoff CT. The St. Croix disaster and the National Disaster Medical System. *Ann Emerg Med.* 1991;20:391–395

Schultz CH, Koenig KL. Earthquakes and the practicing physician. *West J Med.* 1992;157:591

Schultz CH, Koenig KL, Noji EK. A medical disaster response to reduce immediate mortality after an earthquake. *N Engl J Med.* 1996;334: 438–444

Society for Academic Emergency Medicine Disaster Medicine White Paper Subcommittee. Disaster medicine: current assessment and blueprint for the future. *Acad Emerg Med.* 1995;2:1068–1076

Teeter DS. Illnesses and injuries reported at Disaster Application Centers following the 1994 Northridge earthquake. *Mil Med.* 1996;161:526–530

Waeckerle JF. Disaster planning and response. *N Eng J Med.* 1991;324: 815–821

Waeckerle JF, Lillibridge SR, Burkle FM Jr, Noji EK. Disaster medicine: challenges for today. *Ann Emerg Med.* 1994;23:715–718

Appendix 1. Resource Directory

American Red Cross (see also Appendix 2 for list of information available on-line). (Please check your telephone book for your local chapter.) Publications available on request include: Adventures of the Disaster Dudes: A Children's Disaster Preparedness Program; Helping Children Cope with Disaster; Disaster Preparedness and After the Flood coloring books.

Federal Emergency Management Agency
PO Box 70274
Washington, DC 20024
(Catalog of publications available on request)

National Disaster Medical System
   All About Sponsoring a DMAT
   A Step-by-Step Guide to Organizing a DMAT
Telephone: (800) 872-6367

American Civil Defense Association
PO Box 910
Starke, FL 32091

Center for Mental Health, Studies of Emergencies
National Institute of Mental Health
US Public Health Service
5600 Fishers Lane, Room 6C-12
Rockville, MD 20857

Disaster Preparedness Office
National Weather Service
8060 13th Street
Silver Spring, MD 20910

Disaster Research Center
Publication List
University of Delaware
Newark, DE 19716

Governor's Office of Emergency Services
Office of Information and Public Affairs
2800 Meadowview Road
Sacramento, CA 95832
Telephone: (916) 262-1843

Community Preparedness Unit
Disaster Preparedness Division
Los Angeles City Fire Department
543 East Edgeware Road
Los Angeles, CA 90026

Citizens of Oakland Respond to Emergencies (CORE)
475 14th Street, 9th Floor
Oakland, CA 94612

Neighborhood Emergency Response Team Training
San Francisco Fire Department
260 Golden Gate Avenue
San Francisco, CA 94102

Aaron T. Ebata, PhD
University of Illinois at Urbana-Champaign
905 South Goodwin Avenue
Urbana, IL 61801
   Children, Stress, and Natural Disasters: A Guide for Teachers
   Children, Stress, and Natural Disasters: School Activities for
     Teachers

Independent Living Resource Center San Francisco
70 10th Street
San Francisco, CA 94103
Telephone: (415) 863-1290, TTY (415) 863-1367
Fax: (415) 863-1290

Appendix 2. Disaster-Related Brochures and Pamphlets from the American Red Cross

Publication	English	Spanish	PDF*
General Preparedness			
Your Family Disaster Plan	X		X
Disaster Supplies Kit	X		X
Emergency Preparedness Checklist	X		X
Helping Children Cope with Disaster	X		
A Checklist for People with Mobility Problems	X	X	X
Disaster Preparedness for Seniors by Seniors	X		
Pets and Disasters: Get Prepared	X		
Food and Water	X		X
Against the Wind: Protecting Your Home from Hurricane Wind Damage	X		X
Disaster Preparedness Coloring Book	X		X
After a Flood... The First Steps	X		X
Disaster Preparedness for People with Disabilities Booklet (PDF File)	X		X
Disaster Preparedness for People with Disabilities (WordPerfect downloadable version)	X		X
Information by Disaster			
Chemical Emergencies	X		
Volcano Emergency Information			X
Are You Ready for a Residential Fire?	X	X	

*PDF (an Adobe format that delivers printed material to your Internet browser). If you do not already have it, download the Acrobat Reader from the Adobe site.

Appendix 2. *(continued)*

Publication	English	Spanish	PDF*
Are You Ready for a Flood or a Flash Flood?	X		
Are You Ready for a Hurricane?	X	X	
Are You Ready for a Heat Wave?	X	X	
Are You Ready for an Earthquake?	X	X	
Are You Ready for a Tornado?	X	X	
Are You Ready for a Thunderstorm?	X	X	
Are You Ready for a Wildfire?	X		
Are You Ready for a Winter Storm?	X	X	

Appendix 3. Available Disaster-Related Web Sites

www.Usatoday.Com/Weather
www.Ag.Uiuc.Edu/Disaster/Csndactx
www.Co.Sacramento.Ca.Us/Emergenc.Ops/Fameq
www.Slonent.Org/Pv/Ipoes/Oeslist
www.Losaltosonline.Com/Earthq
www.Redcross.Org/Disaster/Safety
www.Fema.Gov
www.Sema.State.Mo.Us/
www.Disaster.Org
www.Yahoo.Com/Environment_&_Nature/Disasters
www.Eas.Slu.Edu/Earthquake_Center

Appendix 4. State Emergency Management Directors

Director
Alabama Emergency Management Agency
5898 County Road 41
PO Drawer 2160
Clanton, AL 35045-5160
Telephone: (205) 280-2201
Fax: (205) 280-2410
State World Wide Web Internet address:
http://alaweb.asc.edu/govern.html

Director
Alaska Division of Emergency Services
PO Box 5750
Fort Richardson, AK 99505-5750
Telephone: (907) 428-7039
Fax: (907) 428-7009
State World Wide Web Internet address: http://www.state.ad.us

Director
Arkansas Office of Emergency Services
PO Box 758
Conway, AR 72033
Telephone: (501) 329-5601
Fax: (501) 327-8047
State World Wide Web Internet address: http://www.state.ar.us

Director
California Office of Emergency Services
2800 Meadowview Road
Sacramento, CA 95832
Telephone: (916) 262-1816
Fax: (916) 262-1677
State World Wide Web Internet address:
http://www.oes.ca.gov:8001/

Director
Colorado Office of Emergency Management
Division of Local Government
Department of Local Affairs
15075 South Golden Road
Golden, CO 80401-3979
Telephone: (303) 273-1622
Fax: (303) 273-1795
State World Wide Web Internet address:
http://www.state.co.us/gov_dir/loc_affairs_dir/oem.htm

Director
Connecticut Office of Emergency Management
Department of Public Safety
360 Broad Street
Hartford, CT 06105
Telephone: (203) 566-4343
Fax: (203) 247-0664
State World Wide Web Internet address: http://www.state.ct.us

Director
Delaware Emergency Management Agency
PO Box 527
Delaware City, DE 19706
Telephone: (302) 834-4531
Fax: (302) 326-6045
E-mail: jmulhern@state.de.us
State World Wide Web Internet address:
http://www.state.de.us/govern/agencies/pubsafe/dema
/indxdema.htm

Director
DC Office of Emergency Preparedness
2000 14th Street NW, 8th Floor
Washington, DC 20009
Telephone: (202) 727-6161
Fax: (202) 673-2290
No World Wide Web Internet address

Director
Florida Division of Emergency Management
2740 Centerview Drive
Tallahassee, FL 32399-2100
Telephone: (904) 413-9969
Fax: (904) 488-1016
E-mail: myersj@dca.state.fl.us
State World Wide Web Internet address:
http://www.scri.fsu.ed/pasko/fem/plans.html

Director
Georgia Emergency Management Agency
PO Box 18055
Atlanta, GA 30316-0055
Telephone: (404) 624-7000
Fax: (404) 635-7205
State World Wide Web Internet address: http://www.state.ga.us

Vice Director
Hawaii State Civil Defense
3949 Diamond Head Road
Honolulu, HI 96816-4495
Telephone: (808) 734-2161
Fax: (808) 733-4287
E-mail: rprice@pdc.org
State World Wide Web Internet address:
http://www.hawaii.gov/gov/

State Director
Idaho Bureau of Disaster Services
4040 Guard Street, Building 600
Boise, ID 83705-5004
Telephone: (208) 334-3460
Fax: (208) 334-2322
E-mail: jcline@bds.state.id.us
State World Wide Web Internet address: http://www.state.id.us

Director
Illinois Emergency Management Agency
110 East Adams Street
Springfield, IL 62702
Telephone: (217) 782-2700
Fax: (217) 785-6043
State World Wide Web Internet address: http://www.state.il.us

Director
Indiana Emergency Management Agency and Department
    of Fire and Building Services
302 West Washington Street, Room E-208
Indianapolis, IN 46204-2760
Telephone: (317) 231-3980
Fax: (317) 232-3895
State World Wide Web Internet address: http://www.state.in.us

Administrator
Iowa Division of Emergency Management
Department of Public Defense
Des Moines, IA 50319
Telephone: (515) 281-3231
Fax: (515) 281-7539
E-mail: dsanders@max.state.ia.us
State World Wide Web Internet address: http://www.state.ia.us

Deputy Director
Kansas Division of Emergency Preparedness
2800 SW Topeka Boulevard
Topeka, KS 66611-1287
Telephone: (913) 274-1401
Fax: (913) 274-1426
E-mail: genek@agtop.wpo.state.ks.us
State World Wide Web Internet address: http://www.state.ks.us

Executive Director
Kentucky Disaster and Emergency Services
EOC Building
Boone National Guard Center
Frankfort, KY 40601-6168
Telephone: (502) 564-8682
Fax: (502) 564-8614
E-mail: padgett@kydes.dma.state.ky.us
State World Wide Web Internet address: http://www.state.ky.us

Assistant Director
Louisiana Office of Emergency Preparedness
PO Box 44217
Baton Rouge, LA 70804
Telephone: (504) 342-1583
Fax: (504) 342-5471
E-mail: sburr@hotmail.com
State World Wide Web Internet address: http://www.state.1a.us

Director
Maine Emergency Management Agency
State Office Building, Station 72
Augusta, ME 04333
Telephone: (207) 287-4080
Fax: (207) 287-4079
E-mail: john.w.libby@state.me.us
State World Wide Web Internet address:
http://www.state.me.us/mema/memahome.htm

Director
Maryland Emergency Management Agency
2 Sudbrook Lane, East
Pikesville, MD 21208
Telephone: (410) 486-4422
Fax: (410) 486-1867
E-mail: dmcmillion@mema.state.md.us
State World Wide Web Internet address:
http://www.maryland.umd.edu/

Director
Massachusetts Emergency Management Agency
400 Worcester Road
PO Box 1496
Framingham, MA 01701-0317
Telephone: (508) 820-2010
Fax: (508) 727-4764
E-mail: drodham_EPS@state.ma.us
State World Wide Web Internet address:
http://www.state.ma.us

Deputy State Director
Michigan Division of Emergency Management
300 South Washington Square, Suite 300
Lansing, MI 48913
Telephone: (517) 334-5103
Fax: (517) 333-4987
State World Wide Web Internet address:
http://www.migov.state.mi.us/

Director
Minnesota Division of Emergency Management
Department of Public Safety
B-5, State Capitol
75 Constitution Avenue
St. Paul, MN 55155-1001
Telephone: (612) 296-0450
Fax: (612) 296-0459
State World Wide Web Internet address:
http://www.state.mn.us-156.98.194.206

Director
Mississippi Emergency Management Agency
PO Box 4501
Fondren Station
Jackson, MS 39296-4501
Telephone: (601) 352-9100
Fax: (601) 352-8314
E-mail: mema@sun1.its.state.ms.us
State World Wide Web Internet address: http://www.state.ms.us

Director
Missouri Emergency Management Agency, PO Box 116
2302 Militia Drive
Jefferson City, MO 65102
Telephone: (314) 526-9146
Fax: (314) 634-7966
E-mail: mosema@mai.state.mo.us
State World Wide Web Internet address:
http://www.dps.state.mo.us

Administrator
Montana Division of Disaster and Emergency Services
1100 North Main
PO Box 4789
Helena, MT 59604-4789
Telephone: (406) 444-6911
Fax: (406) 444-6965
State World Wide Web Internet address: http://www.mt.gov

Assistant Director
Nebraska State Civil Defense Agency
National Guard Center
1300 Military Road
Lincoln, NE 68508-1090
Telephone: (402) 471-7410
Fax: (402) 471-7433
E-mail: krogman@nrcdec.nrc.state.ne.us
State World Wide Web Internet address: http://www.state.ne.us/

Chief
Nevada Division of Emergency Management
Capitol Complex
2525 South Carson Street
Carson City, NV 89710
Telephone: (702) 687-4989
Fax: (702) 687-6788
E-mail: bowen@sierra.net
No World Wide Web Internet address

Deputy State Director
New Jersey Office of Emergency Management
PO Box 7068, Old River Road
West Trenton, NJ 08628-0068
Telephone: (609) 538-6050
Fax: (609) 538-0345
No World Wide Web Internet address

Director
New Mexico Division of Emergency Management
Department of Public Safety
PO Box 1628
Santa Fe, NM 87504-1628
Telephone: (505) 827-9222
Fax: (505) 827-3456
State World Wide Web Internet address:
http://www.129.121.253.22/Index.Htm

Director
New York State Emergency Management Office
22 Security Building, State Campus
Albany, NY 12226-5000
Telephone: (518) 457-9996
Fax: (518) 457-9995
State World Wide Web Internet address:
http://unix2.nysed.gov/ils/

Director
North Carolina Division of Emergency Management
116 West Jones Street
Raleigh, NC 27603
Telephone: (919) 733-3718
Fax: (919) 733-5406
State World Wide Web Internet address: http://www.state.nc.us

Director
North Dakota Division of Emergency Management
PO Box 5511
Bismarck, ND 58502-5511
Telephone: (701) 328-3300
Fax: (701) 328-2119
E-mail: msmail.doug@raneh.state.nd.us
State World Wide Web Internet address: http://www.state.nd.us

Deputy Director
Ohio Emergency Management Agency
2825 West Dublin Granville Road
Columbus, OH 43235-2206
Telephone: (614) 889-7150
Fax: (614) 889-7183
State World Wide Web Internet address: http://www.state.oh.us

Director
Oklahoma Department of Civil Emergency Management
PO Box 53365
Oklahoma City, OK 73152
Telephone: (405) 521-2481
Fax: (405) 521-4053
State World Wide Web Internet address: http://www.state.ok.us

Director
Oregon Division of Emergency Management
595 Cottage Street NE
Salem, OR 97310
Telephone: (503) 378-2911, extension 225
Fax: (503) 588-1378
State World Wide Web Internet address:
http://www.das.state.or.us/oem/oem.htm

Director
Pennsylvania Emergency Management Agency
PO Box 3321
Harrisburg, PA 17105-3321
Telephone: (717) 783-8016
Fax: (717) 651-7800
No World Wide Web Internet address

Director
Rhode Island Emergency Management Agency
State House, Room 27
Providence, RI 02903-1197
Telephone: (401) 421-7333
Fax: (401) 944-1891
State World Wide Web Internet address:
http://www.ids.net/ri/ri.html

Director
South Carolina Emergency Preparedness Division
Office of the Adjutant General
1429 Senate Street
Columbia, SC 29201
Telephone: (803) 734-8020
Fax: (803) 734-8062
E-mail: mckinney@strider.epdstate.sc.us
State World Wide Web Internet address: http://www.state.sc.us

Director
South Dakota Division of Emergency Management
500 East Capitol
Pierre, SD 57501-5070
Telephone: (605) 773-3233
Fax: (605) 733-3580
E-mail: garyw@dem.state.sd.us
State World Wide Web Internet address:
http://www.state.sd.us/state/executive/military/military.html

Director
Tennessee Emergency Management Agency
3051 Sidco Drive
PO Box 41502
Nashville, TN 37204-1502
Telephone: (615) 741-6528
Fax: (615) 242-9635
State World Wide Web Internet address: http://www.state.tn.us

State Coordinator
Texas Division of Emergency Management
Department of Public Safety
PO Box 4087, North Austin
Austin, TX 78733-0225
Telephone: (512) 465-2443
Fax: (512) 424-2444
State World Wide Web Internet address:
http://www.texas.gov/agency/405.html

Director
Utah Division of Comprehensive Emergency Management
State Office Building, Room 1110
Salt Lake City, UT 84114
Telephone: (801) 538-3400
Fax: (801) 538-3770
State World Wide Web Internet address: http://www.state.ut.us

Director
Vermont Division of Emergency Management
Waterbury State Complex
103 South Main Street
Waterbury, VT 05671-2101
Telephone: (802) 244-8721
Fax: (802) 244-8655
State World Wide Web Internet address:
http://www.cit.state.vt.us

State Coordinator
Virginia Department of Emergency Services
310 Turner Road
Richmond, VA 23225-6491
Telephone: (804) 674-2497
Fax: (804) 674-2490
State World Wide Web Internet address: http://www.state.va.us

Director
State of Washington
Military Department
Emergency Management Division
PO Box 40955
Olympia, WA 98504-0955
Telephone: (206) 459-9191
Fax: (206) 923-4591
State World Wide Web Internet address:
http://olympus.dis.wa.gov/www/clear.html

State Director
West Virginia Office of Emergency Services
Main Capitol Building, Room EB-80
Charleston, WV 25305-0360
Telephone: (304) 558-5380
Fax: (304) 344-4538
State World Wide Web Internet address:
http://lcweb.loc.gov/global/state/wv-gov.html

Administrator
Wisconsin Division of Emergency Government
2400 Wright Street
PO Box 7865
Madison, WI 53707
Telephone: (608) 242-3232
Fax: (608) 242-3247
State World Wide Web Internet address: http://www.state.wi.us

Coordinator
Wyoming Emergency Management Agency
PO Box 1709
Cheyenne, WY 82003
Telephone: (307) 777-4900
Fax: (307) 635-6017
E-mail: wema@wy-iso.army.mil
State World Wide Web Internet address:
Gopher://ferret.state.wy.us:70/11/wgov%09$

Manager
American Samoa Territorial Emergency Management
  Coordination
Department of Public Safety
PO Box 1086
Pago Pago, AS 96799
Telephone: (011)(684) 633-2331
Fax: (011)(684) 633-2300
No World Wide Web Internet address

Director
Guam Division of Civil Defense Emergency Services Office
PO Box 2877
Agana, GU 96910
Telephone: (011)(671) 477-9841
Fax: (011)(671) 477-3727
World Wide Web Internet address: http://ns.gov.gu/

Civil Defense Coordinator
Mariana Islands Office of Civil Defense
Capitol Hill
Saipan, Mariana Islands 96950
Telephone: (011)(670) 322-9529
Fax: (011)(670) 322-2545
No World Wide Web Internet address

Civil Defense Coordinator
Republic of the Marshall Islands
PO Box 15
Majuro, Republic of the Marshall Islands 96960
Telephone: (011)(692) 730-3232
Fax: (011)(692) 625-3649
No World Wide Web Internet address

Special Assistant to the President of Micronesia Disaster
  Coordination
Office of the President
PO Box 490
Kolonia, Pohnpei-Micronesia 96941
Telephone: (011)(691) 320-2822
Fax: (011)(691) 320-2785
No World Wide Web Internet address

Palau NEMO Coordinator
Office of the President
PO Box 100
Koror, Republic of Palau 96940
Telephone: (011)(680) 488-2422
Fax: (011)(680) 488-3312
No World Wide Web Internet address

Director
Puerto Rico Civil Defense Agency
Office of the Governor
PO Box 5127
San Juan, PR 00906
Telephone: (809) 724-0124
Fax: (809) 725-4244
No World Wide Web Internet address

Deputy Director
Virgin Islands Office of Civil Defense and Emergency Services
102 Estate Atmon
St. Croix, VI 00820
Telephone: (809) 773-2244
Fax: (809) 774-1491
No World Wide Web Internet address

Delivering Pediatric Emergency Care in Rural Communities

Key Points About Pediatric Emergency Care in Rural Communities

1. The primary-care pediatrician is an important physician of care.
2. Emergency telephone notification systems vary greatly.
3. Links to higher levels of care with pediatric receiving facilities are important.
4. A system for interfacility transport should be in place.

Introduction

The rural pediatric primary-care physician may be much more aware of the need for a system for delivering emergency care to children than the urban counterpart. The rural physician may often be requested to assume a role in the organization of emergency medical services for children (EMS-C). In this role, the physician should address each of the important components of EMS-C (see Chapter 14). These interrelated components are known as the "EMS-C continuum of care." A multifaceted approach to the EMS-C continuum is necessary to ensure optimal outcome for children who experience emergencies. In this chapter, each of the components will be presented in reference to the rural practitioner.

Primary Injury Prevention

The rural primary-care physician is well positioned to lead community injury-prevention activities. The physician is generally well respected in the community and has experience and knowledge of the ill effects of childhood injuries. Epidemiology of rural injury may vary from national trends. Intentional injury is more likely to be due to abuse of children by adults rather than to gang violence. Farm injuries to children also are important. Drowning may occur in streams or quarries rather than home swimming pools. Prevention programs should be included to reduce motor-vehicle occupant, pedestrian, bicycle, and farm injuries and injuries from burns and falls. Local activities should be community driven by using local data to target prevalent injuries. Emergency department surveillance may be a source of important data. A useful resource is the AAP book *Injury Prevention and Control for Children and Youth*. The interested physician will want to become familiar with the AAP TIPP (The Injury Prevention Program) and the National Safe Kids Program. The use of educational programs that are readily available and that have been validated in the field saves times and ensures effective intervention strategies. In well-child visits, offer anticipatory guidance that includes injury prevention information and instruction for parents and children in accessing emergency services.

Emergency Notification

Emergency notification systems include 911 system capabilities. Enhanced 911 that identifies the caller's location is more expensive and may not be in place in the rural setting. The 911 center may or may not provide prearrival instructions to callers. If the local community does not have true 911 services, dialing "911" may result in connection to an operator two states away. Educate families in the proper use of the local emergency notification system. The AAP First-Aid Chart has a space for families to record non-911 emergency numbers. Educational materials for training young children such as the NHTSA (National Highway Traffic Safety Administration) Make the Right Call program are available on loan from many state EMS offices. A number of states now have EMS-C offices that can assist local communities in obtaining such educational programs (see Chapter 3). The National EMS-C Resource Center has a clearinghouse function for all EMS-C products.

The rural primary-care physician may be called on to assist the local emergency notification center in developing policy and protocols for handling pediatric emergencies. The physician may also be called on to assist community public service and public health professionals in advocating for a 911 program. Assistance from a state or regional AAP chapter or COPEM (Committee on Pediatric Emergency Medicine) may prove invaluable in assisting in the development of EMS-C in a rural community.

Emergency Information Form and Children With Special Healthcare Needs

Children with special healthcare needs (CSHCN), especially technology-dependent children, are now a focus of national attention. These children present a special challenge to the rural physicians because the pediatric subspecialists are not readily available. The AAP-ACEP (American College of Emergency Physicians) Emergency Information Form (EIF) may be especially useful for these children. The EIF is a one-page (front-back) summary of the child's medical status that can be given to parents, the local EMS, local emergency departments, and schools. Because rural communities are small, it may be easier to develop individual healthcare plans for CSHCN. Some EMS systems are beginning to include an EMS home visit to these children as part of the initiation of a local special-needs EIF program (see Chapter 15).

Out-of-Hospital

Training

Assist local EMS in training for pediatric emergency care. Pediatric patients are typically responsible for 10% of ambulance calls. The percentage may be significantly less in rural communities. Rural EMS squads are often composed of volunteers or mixed volunteer-paid staff. Many rural hospitals are not routinely staffed by board-prepared emergency physicians, and the local pediatrician can be a consultant for the management of pediatric emergencies. The pediatrician is a valuable resource to the local EMS in the training of personnel in the areas of normal child development, behavior, and physiology. Take the AAP-American Heart Association Pediatric Advanced Life Support (PALS) course to become familiar with the training and backgrounds of out-of-hospital and emergency department colleagues, to facilitate interactions with out-of-hospital personnel, and to maintain familiarity with pediatric resuscitation drugs and protocols. Minimize liability risk by maintaining PALS training. The rural physician is an invaluable training resource for out-of-hospital providers. Become a PALS instructor or Neonatal Resuscitation

Program (NRP) instructor to help improve pediatric resuscitation skills in the community. Participate in Advanced Pediatric Life Support: the Pediatric Emergency Medicine Course, jointly sponsored by AAP and the ACEP (see Chapter 2).

Medical Direction

Medical supervision of EMS systems has two components: on-line and off-line medical direction. All advanced out-of hospital providers must function under the direction of a physician— usually a squad or county medical director. The care delivered is prescribed by protocol, which often requires direct on-line approval by a physician of procedures and medication administration. This approval is often arranged through a regional EMS medical command center. The off-line medical direction is multifaceted and includes protocol development, quality assurance, and recertification of physicians. The off-line medical direction functions are usually reviewed at a local community, regional, or state level. Whenever possible, participate in these review committees and help to form an EMS-C committee. Most AAP chapters now have a COPEM that can provide expert help in protocol development and other off-line medical-direction functions. Rural states generally rely on pediatricians for their state COPEM. When these committees are requested to help develop policy, they can obtain assistance, if needed, from the AAP national COPEM.

Emergency Department Care

The staffing of emergency departments can vary from triage by a nurse or physician assistant supported by rotating family physician backup to 24-hour staffing by several fellowship-trained pediatric emergency physicians. The rural community hospital is most likely to be staffed by rotating physicians who may or may not stay in the hospital during the shift. A recent Consumer Product Safety Commission survey suggested that only 61% of hospitals had pediatric consultation available at all times for the emergency department. A pediatrician who cannot contribute to other EMS-C efforts can make a significant contribution by serving as an on-call person for the local emergency department. Other important pediatric functions in the emergency department include participation in quality improvement, trauma reviews, death reviews, disaster planning, equipment and physical plant planning, and fundraising for pediatric equipment and space in the emergency department (see Chapter 10).

The AAP is currently working with the ACEP and many other groups through the Health Resources and Services Administration (HRSA), Maternal and Child Health Bureau, to develop a set of minimum pediatric emergency department standards. The new minimal standards will allow pediatricians and emergency physicians in local communities to advocate with authority for improvements in emergency capability.

Rural Clinics in Communities Without Hospitals

Rural clinics in communities without hospitals need to examine the forthcoming standards for applicability to their clinical settings. The rural pediatrician who must stabilize patients for transport without the support of a local hospital may want to have equipment available equivalent to that of a pediatric standby facility as defined in the 1995 AAP policy. A recent AAP Clinical Quality Improvement Program (ACQIP) study suggested that approximately 58% of pediatricians have suction available in offices, 23% have Magill forceps, 32% have intraosseous needles, and 91% have oxygen available. Obtain these lifesaving pieces of equipment. They are relatively inexpensive.

Interfacility Transport

Interfacility transport is of special importance in rural areas. Requirements to transfer a patient to a facility with a higher level of care are discussed in Chapters 18, 21, and 22. When pediatric transport teams are not available from the tertiary center, the problems become considerably more complex. Training and certification limit the scope of practice for rural EMTs and EMT paramedics during interfacility transport. Such persons must work under the direction of a physician. Nurses working in rural hospitals are limited by their licenses and training in the interhospital transport environment. In addition, many states require that at least one EMT accompany any patient in an emergency vehicle. Only the primary-care or emergency physician possesses the necessary skills, experience, and authority for independent decision making to safely transport a critically ill pediatric patient who has been successfully resuscitated and stabilized in an emergency department or clinic. Discuss the management of pediatric critical care patients with emergency or critical care physicians at the receiving hospital. In extreme weather conditions, the patient may be best managed by the primary-care physician and other staff in the rural hospital, with close interaction by telephone or telemedicine with pediatric subspecialists at a pediatric receiving hospital, without attempts to move the patient until weather conditions improve.

The Receiving Hospital

Investigate the quality of care at pediatric receiving hospitals that serve the area and refer to a center that provides high-quality, family-centered care. Some institutions may have resources for trauma care, whereas others specialize in medical care. Some receiving hospitals have both (see Chapter 12). Compare the receiving hospital's capability with existing standards for level I pediatric emergency centers and AAP and SCCM (Society for Critical Care Medicine) standards for pediatric intensive care units. Inquire about various family experiences at the receiving hospital. Choice of a receiving hospital may need to be based on a site visit. Visit the center(s) where patients are routinely referred.

Some rural states do not have in-state pediatric critical care centers as receiving hospitals. If patients are to be sent out of state, the protocols and procedures may require review by attorneys and government officials in regard to the liability questions concerning transport, care, and reimbursement.

Lack of access to care due to insurance restrictions is a frequently encountered problem. The rural physician can avoid this difficulty by entering into transport agreements with pediatric receiving hospitals that require acceptance of all patients irrespective of physician status. Be especially cognizant of the potential effect of any agreements with managed care organizations on these relations with receiving hospitals (see Chapter 7).

Rehabilitation Services

Rehabilitation services require the same sort of selective review by the primary-care physician as do other services. The rehabilitative services should be available to all patients, irrespective of payer status, and should be responsive to psychosocial and medical as well as rehabilitative needs of the child and family. Rehabilitation services must include return referral to the child's medical home, as well as the medical home's participation.

EMS-C Advocacy by the Medical Home

The rural primary-care physician is uniquely positioned to advocate for EMS-C. The community accepts this physician's judgment and credentials. Advocacy for EMS-C legislation and injury-prevention legislation can be very effective because of the rural physician's relations with patient families who may know lawmakers and with the rural members of the state legislatures. Advocacy for EMS-C might include advocacy for an EMS-C bill or for consideration of EMS-C matters of fiscal and policy plans of local, regional, and state EMS systems (see Chapter 20).

Summary

Most rural practitioners want to be an integral part of the communities that they serve. Awareness of the need for a multifaceted approach to EMS-C will help them to develop an integrated approach for children who require emergency care in the community. Many community needs addressed by the pediatric emergency physician and the pediatric intensive care specialist in urban communities will need to be met by the rural primary-care physician. The AAP offers the following recommendations in its recent policy statement titled "The Role of the Pediatrician in Rural EMS-C":

1. Help organize and continuously participate in an emergency medical services (EMS) community committee responsible for local system design and development, including educational programs, structured protocols, pediatric ready access communication availability (for dispatchers to emergency department physicians), hospital care and transport (with a special focus on long time and distance issues), and continuous reassessment of all procedural matters, data collection, and quality improvement. This system should integrate well with, and be supported by, state EMS.

2. Ensure appropriate pediatric equipment for physician (pediatrician, family practitioner) and other rural healthcare professional (physician assistant, nurse practitioner) offices, transport vehicles, and recipient facilities.
3. Prepare office staff to deal with pediatric emergencies and personally certify in pediatric resuscitation programs [Pediatric Advanced Life Support (PALS), Advanced Pediatric Life Support (APLS), and Neonatal Resuscitation Program (NRP)].
4. Prepare parents and child caretakers to deal with pediatric emergencies.
5. Provide guidance in recruiting and retaining small community out-of-hospital providers and emergency department physicians who have pediatric expertise, and help them maintain skills and comfort with pediatric emergencies by providing sensitive review (eg, critical incident stress debriefing, reassurance), continuing medical education, and pediatric office rotations.
6. Have a mechanism in place for transfer of patients for higher levels of care to pediatric receiving hospitals in the state or, if necessary, out of state.
7. Develop EMS-C legislative agendas.
8. Generate and stimulate community prevention programs.
   The rural pediatrician who wishes to improve EMS-C in his community will most likely be successful by first learning about scope of practice, function, organization, and decision-making in local and regional EMS systems. The rural pediatrician who volunteers to assist with teaching will likely take part in other ways and thus be able to affect the ways in which EMS affect children in the community.

Suggested Reading

American Academy of Pediatrics. *Pediatric Emergency Medical Sevices Act* [Model legislation]. Elk Grove Village, IL: American Academy of Pediatrics; 1994

American Academy of Pediatrics Committee on Accident and Poison Prevention. Rural injuries. *Pediatrics.* 1988;81:902–903

American Academy of Pediatrics Committee on Hospital Care. Facilities and equipment for the care of pediatric patients in a community hospital. *Pediatrics.* 1998;101:1089–1090

American Academy of Pediatrics Committee on Hospital Care and Pediatric Section of the Society for Critical Care Medicine. Guidelines and levels of care for pediatric intensive care units. *Pediatrics.* 1993;92:166–175

American Academy of Pediatrics Committee on Injury and Poison Prevention, Widome MD, ed. *Injury Prevention and Control for Children and Youth,* 3rd ed. Elk Grove Village, IL: American Academy of Pediatrics; 1997

American Academy of Pediatrics Committee on Pediatric Emergency Medicine. Guidelines for pediatric emergency care facilities. *Pediatrics.* 1995;96:526–537

American Academy of Pediatrics Committee on Pediatric Emergency Medicine. The role of the pediatrician in rural EMSC. *Pediatrics.* 1998;101:941–943

Day S, McCloskey K, Orr R, Bolte R, Notterman D, Hackel A. Pediatric interhospital critical care transport: consensus of a national leadership conference. *Pediatrics.* 1991;88:696–704

Hirschfeld JA. Emergency medical services for children in rural and frontier America: diverse and changing environments. *Pediatrics.* 1995;96:179–184

Institute of Medicine, Committee on Pediatric Emergency Medical Services. Durch JS, Lohr KN, eds. *Emergency Medical Services for Children.* Washington, DC: National Academy Press; 1993

Kessler E, Reiff L. *Estimates of Pediatric Care Readiness in US Hospitals with EDs.* Washington, DC: US Consumer Product Safety Commission; 1997

Sacchetti A, Gerardi M, Barkin R, et al. Emergency information form for children with special needs. *Ann Emerg Med.* 1996;28:324–327

Seidel JS, Henderson DP, Ward P, Wayland BW, Ness B. Pediatric prehospital care in urban and rural areas. *Pediatrics.* 1991;88:681–690

US Congress Office of Technology Assessment. *Rural Emergency Medical Services: Special Report.* Washington, DC: US Congress Office of Technology Assessment, Publication No. OTA-H-445; 1989

Vane DW, Shackford SR. Epidemiology of rural traumatic death in children: a population-based study. *J Trauma.* 1995;38:867–870

Wright JS, Champagne F, Dever GE, Clark FC. A comparative analysis of rural and urban mortality in Georgia, 1979. *Am J Prev Med.* 1985;1:22–29

Legal Aspects of the Provision of Emergency Care

Key Legal Aspects to Remember

1. Know consent laws.
2. Be familiar with child maltreatment and family violence statutes.
3. Know the Good Samaritan law.
4. Be familiar with EMTALA legislation and regulations.
5. Know what is used to define an "emergency" in your community.

Introduction

This chapter is intended to provide the primary-care physician an overview of the legal aspects of providing pediatric emergency care. It is not intended to be a source of legal advice concerning specific situations, but rather to educate the pediatrician about relevant federal and state laws and to enable the practitioner to recognize potential legal aspects. It is important to be familiar with the laws of the state and locality, as well as the rules and protocols of the institutions where you practice.

Consider establishing certain office protocols to avoid legal pitfalls, and to advise one's patients and their parents about legal matters that they should consider, particularly those related to consent for treatment.

Consent

When providing pediatric emergency care, understanding the laws regarding consent for medical treatment is very important. Be aware of the consent policies of local emergency departments and create a written policy for the practice setting. The office consent policy should conform to local and state law as well as the nature of the practice. Become familiar with state and local laws regarding the definition of an emergency, emancipated minors, mature minors, and treatment to which minors can consent independently.

Parental consent for medical treatment of a minor is generally required prior to treatment. However, consent may not be required in an emergency situation, for specific medical services, or for minors who are considered *emancipated* or *mature*. Numerous situations arise in which the parent is not available to give consent.

Emergency Care

Generally, parental consent is not required in situations where emergency care is necessary. In most cases, a healthcare physician can proceed with treatment if a delay would endanger the patient's health or physical well being. The definition of an emergency is usually not limited to life- or limb-threatening illnesses. However, the definition differs among states as well as institutions and is often ambiguous. Still, it is important to be familiar with the definition in your state. In many hospitals, one or two licensed physicians must sign a form declaring that the treatment is necessary because an emergency might or does exist.

Performing invasive or irreversible procedures without parental consent probably creates a greater risk of liability than do more benign procedures. If this type of procedure is necessary, obtaining a second opinion is advisable. Here, documentation is especially important. If a parent is not available, record your efforts to contact the parents. After treating a minor under emergency circumstances, attempt to contact the child's parents promptly. It should be noted that failure to treat in an emergency is more likely to lead to a charge of malpractice than treating without consent is likely to lead to a charge of battery.

Nonemergency Care

The primary-care pediatrician may confront a number of situations in which care is sought on an urgent basis by an unaccompanied adolescent or a child accompanied by someone who is not a parent or legal guardian. Some of these situations are discussed herein.

The Adolescent Not Requiring Parental Consent
Adolescents Seeking Certain Service

Under state statutes, healthcare practitioners can provide certain medical services without parental consent. Most states permit minors to consent to treatment for sexually transmitted disease, contraception, alcohol and drug abuse, and, in some states, pregnancy. Some states also allow minors to consent to psychiatric care. Many states now require parental notification when a minor requests termination of a pregnancy or has a complication of a pregnancy. Check your state laws for these requirements.

Emancipated Minors

Parental consent is not required for minors deemed "emancipated." In general, a minor is usually recognized as emancipated if he or she is married, living separately and apart from his or her parents, financially independent, pregnant, a parent, or in the military. Some states specify that runaways can consent to general medical care because these minors live separate and apart from their parents. Minors in boarding schools or camps are usually not considered emancipated. However, persons enrolled in college may be deemed emancipated minors. A judicial order of emancipation can create emancipated minor status.

Once this status is established, in most states, a minor is treated legally as an adult and can consent to his or her medical care; informed consent obtained from the minor should be documented.

Mature Minors

"Mature minors" are deemed capable of making their own medical decisions. A minor is considered mature if he or she demonstrates an ability to make informed decisions and to understand the nature of the proposed treatment as well as its risks and benefits. Some minors may be mature enough to make important decisions about their medical treatment in the eyes of a court or as defined by state law. Typically, a minor deemed "mature" is between 14 and 17 years old. Minors aged 16 to 17 are more likely to be considered mature. Before treating an adolescent minor without parental consent, a physician should consider the age and maturity of the adolescent, the nature of the illness, and the risks of the procedure. The less risky a procedure, the more likely that a minor will be permitted to consent on his or her own. In emergency situations, the minor should sign a consent form for the needed procedures.

Minors Not Accompanied by a Parent

Parental consent is not required in an emergency situation. In situations that require urgent, but nonemergency care, the treating physician may be unsure about whether to proceed with treatment without parental consent, even if the minor is accompanied by another adult, such as a babysitter, coach, or teacher. Failure to evaluate and treat creates the risk of a charge of negligence, whereas treating without consent creates the risk of a charge of battery.

To avoid such dilemmas, it is advisable for the primary-care pediatrician to ask parents or legal guardians to complete general consent forms when they expect to be unavailable. Ask parents to provide forms to the physician's office, schools, day-care centers, camps, and other child care givers, including noncustodial relatives. These forms will generally allow a physician to treat a child for nonemergency conditions, because the adult accompanying the minor acts *in loco parentis*. Model forms are available from numerous medical associations such as the American College of Emergency Physicians (ACEP). In general, these forms should state that the parent consents to care that health practitioners deem necessary. In addition, parents should specify that they consent to the person caring for the minor to arrange for routine or emergency treatment necessary to protect the health of the child. The forms should specify the period for which this consent applies. Parents should include information about the child's allergies, any medication being taken by the child, immunizations, chronic illness, and names of preferred physicians and medical facilities. Encourage parents to become familiar with the consent policies of their child's school and child-care physician. In addition, parents should make sure that their children and children's caretakers know the children's home telephone numbers, the parents' work telephone numbers, and the names of the parents' workplaces.

If the person accompanying a minor is the legal guardian of the child, he or she can usually consent to the treatment. Be sure to note the circumstances in the patient's medical record when a person other than a parent or legal guardian gives consent for treatment of a child. Attach a copy of the consent form, if possible.

Minors in Foster Care

Because of foster-care placement or temporary or permanent kinship care, a child's biological parent may be unavailable to consent. Many state statutes permit foster parents to consent to routine treatment of a minor, including medical, dental, or mental health treatment. Obtain consent from the natural parents if the procedure is considered risky or elective. Again, the patient's medical records should indicate who provided consent. In some states, the officers of the juvenile court and their representatives are the only agents permitted to give consent for medical treatment of children under their jurisdiction.

Minors in Detention Facilities

Generally, routine medical care can be provided to minors in detention facilities. Again, if the treatment is high risk or elective, the healthcare physician should seek parental consent.

Children of Divorced or Separated Parents

When parents are divorced or separated, the custodial parent generally has authority to make treatment decisions for the child without approval of the noncustodial parent.

If a noncustodial parent presents the child, usually possession of the child allows that parent to consent to treatment. (In joint custody arrangements, the same principle applies.) Unfortunately, situations arise when parents disagree about treatment for their child. For patients whose parents are separated or divorced, it may be advisable to discuss medical treatment decision making with parents before an urgent situation arises.

Refusal to Consent to Treatment

In cases in which parents refuse lifesaving treatment for their children, various forms of recourse are available. A physician alone should not override the parents' wishes unless compelled to do so by the medical condition of the child. In a hospital, the physician can turn to the institutional ethics committee, which may be able to resolve treatment disputes without legal intervention. If this route is not available or appropriate (such as in urgent situations), it may be necessary to notify the state's child protective services (CPS) system, which is responsible for investigating and intervening in cases in which a child is thought to be in danger. CPS officials may take custody of the child and consent to treatment on the child's behalf. A judicial hearing is another tool. Courts can order necessary treatment despite the objections of a patient's parents. In addition, a court can authorize a third party to consent to the treatment.

Sometimes, objection to treatment is based on religious grounds. The same courses of action just described are available in such cases. It is not uncommon, for example, for a hospital to seek and be granted a court order for a blood transfusion for a child of parents who object to this procedure on religious grounds. Although most states have *religious exemption* laws shielding parents from liability for religion-based medical neglect, all states receiving federal funds under the Child Abuse Prevention and Treatment Act, or CAPTA (virtually every state receives such funds), are required to have in place mechanisms to ensure that children receive necessary medical care regardless of their parents' religious beliefs. Therefore, pediatricians should pursue legal intervention for children in such situations, even if initially advised that parents' religious beliefs preclude state action.

Child Maltreatment and Domestic Violence

Child Maltreatment

Child abuse and neglect, or child maltreatment, generally refers to physical abuse, sexual abuse, emotional abuse, and neglect. Neglect includes failure to provide clothing, shelter, emotional support, education, and medical or dental care. One study found that about half of all child abuse was some type of orofacial injury. Failure to seek proper dental care for the treatment of caries may result from many factors including neglect. The point at which to consider a parent negligent and to begin intervention occurs after the parent has been properly alerted to the nature and extent of the child's condition, the specific treatment needed, and the mechanism of accessing that neglect.

The definitions of abuse and neglect vary by state, so it is important to know the laws in your jurisdiction. All 50 states, the District of Columbia, Guam, Puerto Rico, and the United States

Virgin Islands require physicians to report suspected child abuse or neglect. Most statutes require that a doctor make a report when there is a reasonable suspicion that a child has been abused. Physicians are considered mandatory reporters. Failure to report can result in civil and criminal action for negligence, substantial fines, or incarceration. The majority of states provide reporters with *good faith immunity,* which insulates them from civil or criminal liability for an error made in good faith. Be aware, however, that state courts differ in their interpretation of reporting statutes, and the good faith provision has been challenged. Some courts apply a subjective test, whereas others use an objective test of a reporter's good faith. A small number of states, including California, offer *absolute immunity* to reporters of abuse or neglect.

All states specify how a person should report child abuse or neglect. Generally, reports are made by telephone to the CPS and detail the age and address of child, the address of the parents, and the type of suspected abuse or neglect. Doctor-patient confidentiality is exempted under these circumstances. In situations where it is necessary to remove the child from the home, hospitalize the child, or protect siblings, social services and the police often intervene. Carefully prepared and detailed written documentation is important and usually mandated by law when reporting child abuse or neglect. Record information about your findings and include any statements made by the parent or the child or both. Communication with the child at an appropriate level is important. Interviews with the child should be conducted alone. Photographs (with notations of time and date taken) of the injuries are useful for documentation of inflicted trauma. Include criteria for obtaining and properly handling laboratory tests, forensic specimens, and photographs in office protocols for child abuse. It may be advisable to consult with specialists in suspected sexual abuse cases or questionable physical abuse cases to ensure that examinations and specimen collection are conducted in the manner necessary to document the case in a legal proceeding. Many municipalities have *centers of excellence* designed specifically for referral of children with suspected physical or sexual abuse. These centers usually have multidisciplinary specialists, including physicians, nurses, psychologists, social workers, and law enforcement personnel who are trained in the collection of forensic evidence. Know where these centers are located in your community and have their telephone numbers available in the office for consultation and referral.

The primary-care physician should be familiar with the indicators of child abuse and neglect, state definitions of child abuse and neglect, how and when to intervene in suspected cases, how to collect and document necessary information and evidence, and where to find expert consultation.

Domestic Violence

Become familiar with the state and local laws and community resources available on suspected domestic violence (spousal, elder abuse) so that you can help victims remove themselves from dangerous situations. Some states do have mandatory reporting of domestic violence.

Elder Abuse

Elder abuse is a common problem and, in many states, is reportable to social services agencies or law enforcement authorities or both. Be aware of the reporting requirements in your state or municipality. Report all suspected elder abuse.

Firearms

Pediatricians should be aware that it is a violation of federal law for a person to possess a firearm if a restraining order is in place against that person or if that person has been convicted of a domestic violence misdemeanor (including criminal convictions related to child abuse or assault against a significant other, whether or not the perpetrator and victim are married). Because it is recommended that pediatricians ask patients and families about the presence of guns in the home, there may be an occasion to inform families of this law in cases where it may be relevant.

Rape, Incest, and Assaults

As in suspected cases of child abuse and neglect, the primary-care pediatrician may confront other injury cases in which there may be legal ramifications with respect to medical observations and information obtained from patients or those accompanying them. Be aware that documentation in such cases is very important and that it may be necessary to photograph injuries, collect specimens in a proper manner, and report the case to CPS workers or law enforcement authorities. Take measures to protect the patient from additional harm or address the patient's and family's psychosocial needs or both.

Liability and License-Related Matters

Standard of Care

Physicians are required to exercise a reasonable degree of care, skill, and diligence used by other members of the profession in good standing under the circumstances. In general, care rendered must be consistent with the national standard of care, based on the appropriate use of available facilities and medical equipment.

Documentation

Detailed, accurate documentation is important in an emergency or urgent situation in case a poor outcome should lead to malpractice litigation. Charting should be done as promptly as possible to preserve and document important details. Notes should include the date and time of the treatment, diagnoses, and rationale for treatment. In addition, the statements of the patient and his or her family should be included when possible. Parental or alternative consent, or the reasons that it was not obtained, should be recorded. Document consultations including requests and times for transfer or transport and the names of the personnel. Document the dates and times of all multiple assessments.

Because it may be difficult to record notes in an emergency medical situation, it is advisable to assign a recorder or use a dictation machine so that accurate notes can be transcribed later. It may be advisable to establish an office protocol for documentation in emergency situations that staff can follow should an emergency arise in your office.

Office Equipment, Protocols, and Staff Training

As stated in Chapter 5, the primary-care physician should ensure that minimum equipment is available in the office, that staff are adequately trained in its use, and that office protocols are in place for handling emergency telephone calls, walk-ins, or situations that arise in the office owing to complications of treatment, deterioration of a patient's condition, choking, or an intentional or unintentional injury. Protocols and staff training and certification should be documented. Pediatricians should also document their education of patients about how emergencies should be handled, especially when the office is closed. Failure to prepare for a foreseeable emergency could expose the pediatrician to liability for negligence (see Chapter 3).

Good Samaritan Statutes

Good Samaritan laws are designed to encourage rescue efforts by protecting the rescuer from liability. In general, these good Samaritan statutes protect physicians who provide medical assistance at the scene of an emergency. However, in many states, a Good Samaritan statute will not protect acts of gross negligence.

Generally, the Good Samaritan protections apply only if the physician provided care without a preexisting duty to render aid. A statute may specify that a physician cannot demand or receive compensation for the services in question. In addition, some states require good faith judgment that immediate medical care was necessary. The standard of care required differs from state to state; some statutes specifically require that assistance be provided with ordinary or reasonable care.

Some states, such as Utah, extend protection to hospital settings. Primary-care physicians should be aware that some state statutes protect only physicians who are licensed in the state where emergency aid is rendered.

Again, check your local and state laws regarding Good Samaritan statutes.

Failure to Provide Care

In general, a physician is not liable for negligence when failing to come to the aid of someone in danger, although some state laws establish an affirmative duty to rescue subject to fines or misdemeanor. Note, however, that a physician may have an ethical duty to provide emergency aid. Although a physician has the right to decide whom to treat, this right does not exist in some emergency situations. The duty of *necessary rescue* requires a physician to render aid if a person has a critical need for professional assistance. Some courts have specified that a physician cannot withdraw care at a critical stage unless a replacement physician exists.

A handful of states, such as Minnesota and Rhode Island, impose a duty to give reasonable emergency assistance if it can be rendered without danger to the person giving the assistance and care is not being provided by others. However, these statutes appear to apply primarily to persons who are not healthcare practitioners.

Other Liability and License-Related Matters

Disasters

In the aftermath of a natural disaster, such as a hurricane or flood, a primary-care pediatrician may wish to volunteer to render nonemergency care to victims. The legal aspects of rendering emergency care in such cases should be no different from those in other emergency situations. Be aware that legal problems may arise when the pediatrician offers other voluntary services. First, medical liability insurance coverage may exclude services for which the physician is not credentialed or which are performed outside of the normal practice settings. Second, most states do not provide an exception to in-state licensure requirements, even for disaster volunteers. (An exception is California, which allows healthcare practitioners licensed in another state or territory of the United States to provide healthcare for which he or she is licensed, if the care is provided during a state of emergency, and immunizes physicians who render services during "a state of emergency or local emergency" at the express or implied request of a state or local official.) Civil liability is generally not covered by malpractice insurance when healthcare physicians are practicing in a locality that is not specifically cited in their malpractice insurance policies. Physicians are covered when operating under the designated legal disaster management team.

Medical Assistance in Airspace

When aiding in air emergencies, state Good Samaritan laws are not likely to be applicable. Currently, no federal law protects people from liability when they provide good faith aid in an emergency situation on an airplane. Additionally, pediatricians should be aware that medical kits aboard airplanes are not currently required to include pediatric equipment. Therefore, if you are officially responsible for a group of children traveling by air (eg, on a school trip), it may be advisable to carry some equipment that would prepare you for an emergency situation. (The same preparation would be advisable in any situation where you are officially responsible for a group of children.)

The Emergency Medical Treatment and Active Labor Act (EMTALA)

EMTALA was passed in response to Congressional concern about hospitals turning away uninsured patients ("patient dumping"). The law applies to all hospitals with emergency departments that participate in the Medicare or Medicaid program (virtually all hospitals with emergency departments) and to individual physicians in those hospitals. The law protects all patients seeking care at those hospitals regardless of their insurance status.

EMTALA has three key requirements. First, the hospital must provide appropriate medical screening to determine if the patient has an emergency medical condition. Appropriate medical screening requires a uniform process in evaluating an emergency department patient regardless of a patient's insurance status. Second, if an emergency condition exists, the hospital must stabilize the patient's condition or transfer the patient to a facility that can provide such treatment if the hospital is unable to do so. Stabilizing treatment is "any treatment necessary to assure, within reasonable medical probability, that no material deterioration of the condition is likely to result from or occur during the transfer of the individual from a facility." This component of the law also includes any pediatrician or other specialist who is on call on an emergency department panel. These specialists are required to comply with EMTALA and provide consultative services when requested by the emergency department. To stabilize patients in active labor the hospital must either deliver the baby or assure a safe transfer to a facility capable of delivering the infant. Third, a hospital may transfer an unstabilized patient under limited circumstances.

If a hospital fails to follow one of these three requirements, it is subject to civil monetary penalties and civil legal action by the patient who was denied care. Although lawsuits by the aggrieved patient cannot be brought against an individual physician, physicians are subject to civil monetary penalties imposed pursuant to action by the US Department of Health and Human Services. The statute provides that any physician "who is responsible for the examination, treatment, or transfer of an individual in a participating hospital" and who "negligently violates" the Act's requirements is subject to a maximum penalty of $50 000. In addition, a physician can be excluded from federal and state healthcare programs if a physician's violation is "gross and flagrant or is repeated."

Numerous ambiguous issues remain regarding the interpretation of EMTALA. Physicians should be aware that this area of law is complicated and that interpretation varies by court.

It is important for physicians to be familiar with the Health Care Financing Administration (HCFA) guidance on the medical screening examination (MSE). An MSE is the process required to reach, within reasonable clinical confidence, the point at which it can be determined whether a medical emergency does or does not exist. Hospitals are obligated to screen patients to determine if an emergency condition exists. The MSE must be the same for all patients regardless of payer status, and the type of MSE will vary from patient to patient. For some patients, the MSE may consist of a brief history and physical examination; other patients may require extensive evaluations including laboratory and radiologic studies. The guidance further notes that medical screening is not an isolated event. It is an ongoing process. The record must reflect continued monitoring according to the patient's needs and must continue until he or she is stabilized and appropriately transferred.

Aspects of Insurance Coverage

Insurance coverage for emergency department visits has become increasingly uncertain as managed-care plans attempt to curtail emergency department use for nonemergency care. If a primary-care pediatrician has been designated by an insurance plan to make determinations about whether a patient should be treated in an emergency department, it is possible that liability could arise for failure to authorize care that later proved to have been necessary. Therefore, it is important to document all the information that was provided by the emergency department in such situations, as well as the rationale for the decision. (Such documentation would also be helpful in justifying authorizations of care later questioned by the insurance company.)

Prior authorization requirements also may pose a dilemma for a pediatrician in an emergency department when an insurance company denies authorization for treatment but the pediatrician believes that the care is necessary. Of course, medical judgment should prevail in such cases, although the hospital, patient, and physician may be denied reimbursement. Be aware that, under current federal law, the health plans themselves are generally not subject to lawsuits by those whom they insure, but the physician may be exposed to liability for failure to treat. (The issue of health plan liability is currently being debated in Congress.)

To prevent reimbursement problems, physicians should discuss insurance policies with their patients and make sure that they are aware of possible limitations in coverage for emergency department use. Specifically, patients should be familiar with their plans' definitions of emergency care, whether prior authorization is required for emergency services, and the extent to which emergency services outside of the physician network are covered (see Chapters 3 and 7).

Patients and pediatricians should also be aware of the appeal processes for coverage denials. Patients may call on physicians for help in resolving disputes with their insurance companies, so it is important to document referrals to emergency departments.

Some common reimbursement principles for emergency department services are considered next.

"Prudent Layperson" Standard

The Medicare and Medicaid programs, health plans subject to state laws in several states (currently about 15), and (as of 1999) the plans participating in the Federal Employees Health Benefit Plan are required to reimburse for emergency department care if the patient presents with symptoms that a "prudent layperson" could reasonably expect to seriously impair one's health.

(Congress is currently debating whether other insurers should be required to follow the "prudent layperson" standard.)

A *prudent layperson* is defined as a person with average knowledge about health and medicine. *Emergency services* are defined as covered inpatient or outpatient services that are furnished by a qualified physician and are necessary to evaluate and stabilize an emergency medical condition.

An *emergency medical condition* is a medical condition "manifesting itself by acute symptoms of sufficient severity including severe pain, such that a 'prudent layperson' who possesses an average knowledge of health and medicine could reasonably expect the absence of immediate medical attention to result in either placing the health of the individual, or with respect to a pregnant woman, the health of the woman or her unborn child, in serious jeopardy, serious impairment to bodily functions, or serious dysfunction of any bodily organ or part."

Even if the final diagnosis suggests that the patient's symptoms did not require emergency care, the plan is still required to cover the cost of services rendered if a "prudent layperson" standard is in effect. Patients should be aware that, in states without this standard, a plan might refuse to cover emergency department services if the plan retrospectively determines that the symptoms or condition did not constitute an emergency.

Reasonableness Standard

In a several states, such as California and Michigan, a reasonableness standard is applied for reimbursement of emergency department services that does not take into consideration the "prudent layperson" definition of an emergency. This standard requires reimbursement for care and services provided for an emergency medical condition, which is defined as a condition that manifests itself by acute symptoms of sufficient severity, such that the absence of immediate medical attention could reasonably be expected to place the patient's health in serious jeopardy, seriously impair bodily functions, or cause serious dysfunction of any bodily organ or part.

Prior Authorization

Some health plans require prior authorization of emergency

department visits (see Chapter 7). Encourage patients to become familiar with their policies and understand what their plans require. Under federal law, Medicare, Medicaid, and federal employee health plans must cover emergency department visits without prior authorization if the "prudent layperson" test is met. A number of states also require health plans to cover emergency services without prior authorization. Even if a plan does not require prior authorization, patients should still promptly notify their plans of the emergency care. Many plans require that patients advise the plans of their emergency care within 24 hours to 72 hours of the visit and often require authorization for any follow-up care. Pediatricians can be very helpful to their patients by reminding them that they may need to notify their insurance plans promptly after an emergency department visit and follow-up care.

Out-of-Network and Nonparticipating Physicians

In some cases, a health plan refuses to cover emergency services provided outside of the plan's network or by a physician who does not participate in the patient's health plan. In addition, some plans require higher copayments for services rendered by a nonparticipant.

Under federal law, Medicaid and Medicare managed-care organizations are required to cover emergency services regardless of whether the emergency-care physician has a contract with the patient's health plan.

In addition, some state legislatures have recently enacted laws that mandate coverage of emergency services provided by a nonparticipating physician. Most state laws allow the most accessible physician to render emergency care, regardless of whether the physician is part of the health plan.

Other Reimbursement Matters

Many states have legislation requiring that all plans licensed in the state reimburse physicians for any and all services rendered pursuant to EMTALA requirements (discussed earlier).

For Medicaid beneficiaries, federal law ensures coverage for emergency services, permits emergency care and services for aliens not admitted for permanent residence, and prohibits state plans from requiring prior authorization for the dispensing of a 72-hour supply of a covered outpatient prescription in an emergency situation.

Laws regarding reimbursement are rapidly being developed and revised. Currently, numerous pieces of legislation are pending on the state and federal level with regard to reimbursement. Keep abreast of changes that affect you and your patients. It is important to encourage patients to review their plans and understand what services are covered. Regardless of coverage, physicians should make clear that patients should utilize the emergency department when necessary.

Summary

There are numerous laws and legal doctrines relevant to the provision of emergency medical services to children. It is advisable for pediatricians to become familiar with state and local laws regarding consent, child abuse and neglect reporting, the definition of an emergency, and Good Samaritan laws, among others. To avoid legal problems in treating children's emergency or urgent medical conditions, it may be advisable (among other measures discussed earlier) for the primary-care pediatrician to:

- establish office protocols for handling emergencies, including methods of documenting referrals, treatment provided, consultation, and calls for transport
- require and document staff training and certification
- advise patients and parents about legal aspects of treatment that they should consider, particularly in relation to consent for treatment, and ask parents or legal guardians to complete general consent forms when they expect to be unavailable
- discuss medical treatment decision making with parents who are separated or divorced
- consult law-enforcement authorities, CPS authorities, or relevant pediatric experts in cases of suspected child abuse or neglect, rape, incest, or assault
- become familiar with federal and state laws regarding insurance coverage for emergency conditions and carefully document referrals to emergency departments and rationale for authorizing or failing to authorize emergency department care for patients

- be familiar with the EMTALA requirements for medical screening, emergency treatment, the requirements for emergency department consultants, and transfer for higher levels of care
- become familiar with the legal recourses and other community resources available to assist persons who you suspect are subjected to domestic violence (spousal, elder abuse), so that you can help them to remove themselves from dangerous situations
- have important telephone numbers readily available in the office such as: EMS, CPS, law enforcement, the juvenile court liaison, hospital ethics committee chair, malpractice insurance agent, the practice attorney, and so forth
- have a protocol for referral of suspected child abuse to a "center of excellence" if one exists in the community or region

Although pediatricians should try to be informed about legal matters, they should not allow legal or reimbursement considerations to impede access to necessary emergency medical services for their patients or others.

Resources
General

State or local medical societies are a potential source of relevant laws affecting practicing physicians. State and local bar associations also may have copies of relevant laws and summaries of case law on certain topics. For laws regarding child-abuse and neglect reporting, a pediatrician can contact the state, county, or city child protective services agency or the National Clearinghouse on Child Abuse and Neglect Information (see subsection titled Child Abuse and Domestic Violence in this Resources section). For laws regarding reproductive health services, local family planning organizations may be able to provide relevant laws.

Many state and federal laws are posted on the Internet, although it is important to confirm that these versions are up-to-date.

Consent

American Academy of Pediatrics Committee on Pediatric Emergency Medicine. Consent for medical services for children and adolescents. *Pediatrics*. 1993;92: 290–291. Also available on the Web at: http://www.aap.orgpolicy/04481.html

American Academy of Pediatrics Committee on Bioethics. Informed consent, parental permission, and assent in pediatric practice. *Pediatrics*. 1995;95:314–317. Also available on the Web at: http://www. aap.org/policy/00662.html

American Academy of Pediatrics Committee on School Health. Guidelines for urgent care in school. *Pediatrics*. 1990;86:999–1000. Also available on the Web at: http://www.aap.org/policy/03376.html

American Academy of Pediatrics Task Force on Adolescent Assault Victim Needs. Adolescent assault victim needs: a review of issues and a model protocol. *Pediatrics*. 1996;98:991–1001. Also available on the Web at: http://www.aap.org/policy/00991.html

American College of Emergency Physicians. Consent form available. Send self-addressed, stamped envelope to: 900 17th Street, NW, Suite 1250, Washington, DC 20006. Attn: Public Relations Department. Also available on-line at http://www.acep.org

Issues in Brief: Teenagers' Right to Consent to Reproductive Health Care. The Alan Guttmacher Institute (1998). Available on the Web at: http://www.agi-usa.org/pubs/ib21.html

Issues in Brief: Lawmakers Grapple with Parents' Role in Teen Access to Reproductive Health Care. The Alan Guttmacher Institute (1995). Available on the Web at: http://206.215.210.5/pubs/ib6.html

Child Abuse and Domestic Violence

National Clearinghouse of Child Abuse and Neglect. Telephone: (800) 394-3366 or (703) 385-7565); E-mail: nccanch@calib.com; Web site: http://www.calib.com/nccanch. (Can provide federal and state statutes regarding mandatory reporting, immunity, penalties for failure to report, definitions of abuse and neglect. All posted on Web site.)

Guidry HM. Childhood sexual abuse. *Am Fam Physician*. 1995;51: 407–414.

Steiner RP, Vansickle K, Lippman SB. Domestic violence: do you know when and how to intervene? *Postgrad Med*. 1996;100:103–116

Liability

American Academy of Pediatrics Committee on Pediatric Emergency Medicine. The pediatrician's role in disaster preparedness. *Pediatrics*. 1997;99:130–133. Also available on the Web at: http://www.aap.org/policy/re9702.html

American Academy of Pediatrics Committee on Hospital Care. Precertification process. *AAP News*. 1992;8:15. Also available on the Web at: http://www.aap.org/policy/619.html

Frey V. The scope of Good Samaritan legislation. *Med Trial Tech Q*. 1993;40:159–169

Furrow B. Forcing rescue: the landscape of health care physician obligations to treat patients. *Health Matrix*. 1993;3:31–87

EMTALA

42 US Code §1395dd (1998)

American College of Emergency Physicians: web page- www.acep.org

Reimbursement

Letters to Health Care Financing Administration (HCFA) regarding the Emergency Service Provision of the Balanced Budget Act of 1997 (advice to parents about selecting health plan) available on the Internet at: http://www.acep.org/policy/ac302000.html.

Health policy tracking service available on the Web at: http://www.hpts. org/HPTS97/home.nsf

Chapter 19

Emergencies at School

Key Points About Emergencies at School

1. Emergencies are common occurrences.
2. They are usually managed by the school nurse or administrative personnel.
3. Primary care physicians should forge linkages with the school health system.
4. Develop plans for CSHCN at school.

Introduction

Very little information exists about the exact nature and frequency of emergencies that occur in or around schools. There is a lack of operational definitions of what constitutes a school injury. The lack of these data in all states has made it difficult for schools, communities, and governments to determine the resources needed to provide optimal emergency care to children in schools. We do know that the school nurse provides most of the healthcare in the school setting. The most common activities performed by the school nurse include: first aid and emergency treatment, immunizations, and vision, hearing, and scoliosis screening. School nurses also coordinate health assessments for children with special healthcare needs (CSHCN).

Only an estimated 26 000 school nurses practice in the 89 000 schools that constitute the elementary and secondary school system in the United States. Although some nurses may be employed at multiple sites, there are still large gaps in coverage. The major professional organization representing school nurses is the National Association of School Nurses (NASN). A 1993 survey conducted by NASN showed that the nurse-to-pupil ratio was the number one area of concern by respondents. In fact, more than one-third of nurses indicated that there was pressure from school administrators to delegate nursing functions to unlicensed personnel.

A shortage of school nurses or lack of school-based health programs may severely affect the management of emergencies.

How prepared are schools and school nurses to manage emergencies? Are services sufficient to manage a range of problems from minor playground injuries to an episode of severe respiratory distress? How well established are the linkages between school health services, emergency medical services (EMS), hospital emergency departments, and primary-care physicians? This chapter explores these questions and offers some guidance for the development or improvement of school emergency services.

Types of School Emergencies

Only limited research has been published on the type of emergencies that arise at school. The few studies available are based on self-reported data and are subject to significant underreporting bias. A survey of Pennsylvania school nurses in 1994 provided a summary of emergencies in schools and included treatment of suicide (46%), drug or alcohol overdose (14%), anaphylaxis (13%), miscarriages (7%), aspiration (3.2%), hemorrhages (4%), and loss of tracheostomy access (0.4%). Only 50% of the surveys were returned, and it was not known how schools routinely tracked and categorized health visits.

A random sample survey of 10% of all school districts in the United States in 1996 reported that the most significant health problems encountered by school health personnel ranged widely from behavioral disturbances to dental problems (Table 25). The same survey examined the provision of school health services by category of physician. Services that might typically be needed in an emergency, such as the administration of first aid, the evaluation of suspected child abuse, the evaluation of behavioral problems, the monitoring of vital signs, and the administration of medications and oxygen, were often performed by school health assistants, clerks, or paraprofessionals, not nurses. In fact, nonnurses performed first aid 57% of the time, indicating the absence of school nurses at many sites.

An earlier survey of more than 200 schools in 1994 looked at current school health services, at the interest in expanding school health services, and at the barriers encountered in the delivery of these services. Of the 111 respondents, only 75% of the schools had access to school nursing services, whereas 33% had no school nurse on site. School nurse availability was on a daily (50%), weekly (32%), biweekly (4%), and monthly (11%) basis. Only 23% of respondents indicated the ability to provide acute care. Perceived barriers to the provision of school health services most often cited by respondents were transportation and funding (Table 26).

Table 25.

Significant Health Problems Encountered by School Personnel

••

Accidents and injuries
Chronic diseases
Communicable diseases
High-risk social behaviors
Lack of access to healthcare
Poverty
Self-esteem problems
Special health needs
Unhealthy life-style habits

••

Source: Modified from Fryer GE, Igoe JB. Functions of school nurses and health assistants in U.S. school health programs. *J Sch Health.* 1996;66:55–58.

Table 26.

Perceived Barriers to Schools Providing and Families Accessing School Health Services

••

Percentage of schools reporting (N = 107)

Barrier	Schools	Families
Limited space	21	6
Limited services	28	25
Transportation	15	70
Insurance	6	26
Funding	63	60
Awareness	33	47
Opposition	19	1

••

Source: Modified from Heneghan AM, Malakoff ME. Availability of school health services for young children. *J Sch Health.* 1997;67:327–332.

A recent study in Utah between 1990 and 1997 found that there were 60 053 injuries statewide at schools. The annual injury rate was 13.7 per 1000 students per year. Of these injuries, at least half resulted in a half-day absence from school or required medical attention. The highest percentage of injuries was among fifth and sixth graders; 4.2% had repeated injuries. The most common contributing factors included collision, tripping, and falls. And most injuries occurred during physical education and recess. The most common serious injuries were fractures (30%), lacerations (24.6%), and sprains (12%).

No study to date has systematically and accurately assessed the patterns of illness and injuries that occur at schools. There are, however, many anecdotal reports, which describe the spectrum of emergency problems. The list includes lacerations, fractures, sprains, bruises, vomiting, fainting, shortness of breath, wheezing, chest pain, amenorrhea, skin rashes, and allergic reactions. The Principle School Disciplinarian Survey on School Violence documented the number of violent crimes taking place in public schools in the 1996–1997 school year. This survey demonstrated an increased prevalence of violent acts taking place in schools. Despite the paucity of data, it is reasonable to assume that the spectrum of childhood illnesses and injuries encountered elsewhere are likely to happen in schools as well.

Emergency Preparedness of Schools

The National Association of State School Nurse Consultants (NASSNC), one of the five member organizations of the National Nurses Coalition of School Health (Figure 24) has written a position paper stating that school nursing services should be provided to all students. The list of recommended services includes the provision of emergency care defined as follows:

1. Assessment, planning, and intervention for emergency management of a student with chronic or debilitating health impairment.
2. Provision of urgent emergency care, to include nursing assessment and emergency response treatment, such as cardiopulmonary resuscitation (CPR), oxygen administration, seizure care, administration of emergency medication, and triage.

3. Postemergency assessment and the development of a preventive action plan.

In 1995, a comprehensive curriculum and training program titled School Nurse Emergency Medical Services for Children (SNEMS-C) was developed through financial support from an EMS-C grant program in Connecticut through the federal Maternal and Child Health Bureau. The objective was to create a program for school nurses to prepare them to manage emergencies in school. To date, the project has produced an instructional manual for school nurses and instructional materials to be used in a trainer-type format. It is the most comprehensive educational tool available for this purpose. From 1995 to 1997, nearly 200 school nurses participated in SNEMS-C pilot programs. The formal course has been offered to more than 1000 school nurses throughout the United States. The content of the curriculum is in accordance with generally accepted standards of practice and is a useful tool in guiding the development of local school policy and practice.

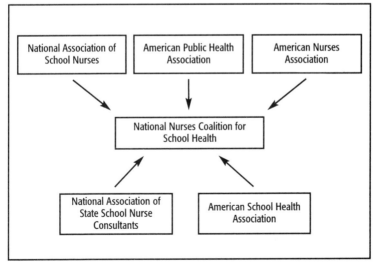

Fig 24. Organizations of the National Nurse Coalition for School Health.

School nurses should initiate comprehensive planning for the management of emergencies at school by emphasizing the need for collaboration and communication with school officials, the community EMS system, parents, and healthcare physicians and facilities. This activity should begin with an assessment of who, what, where, when, and how students might become ill or injured. A written plan is preferred. Table 27 lists the components of a comprehensive school emergency action plan.

Equipment and Resources

Although the level of emergency equipment will vary from school to school on the basis of available resources and the characteristics of the student population, all schools should strive to maintain the basic supplies needed in an emergency. A list of suggested items to be included in a school nurse emergency kit can be found in Table 28.

Table 27.

Components of a School Emergency Action Plan

1. Specific details for calling EMS
2. Notification of school staff of duties in response to an emergency
3. Notification of parent, guardian, or caretaker
4. Standing orders or protocols to be followed
5. Emergency supplies or kits available and easily located
6. Transport protocols
7. Accident or incident reports
8. Follow-up or debriefing after major incident

Note: For more details, see Brainerd EF, ed. SNEMS-C *School Nurse Emergency Medical Services for Children Program School Nurse Manual.* University of Connecticut, Department of Pediatrics. Project MCH 094002-01-0. Washington, DC: Emergency Medical Services for Children, Health Resources Services Administration, Department of Health and Human Services; 1996

Table 28.

School Nurse Emergency Kit Suggested Items (National Association of School Nurses)

Quantity	Item
1	Rescue bag (sufficient space for listed supplies)
3 pairs	Latex gloves (vinyl *preferred* owing to latex allergy)
1	Mouth-to-mask resuscitator (one-way valve)
1*	Disposable bag-mask resuscitator (optional with O_2)
1 pair	Protective eyeglasses
1	Disposable protective gown or apron
1 pair of each	Bandage scissors and EMS scissors
1 each	Blood pressure cuff (adult, child, and extra large)
1	Stethoscope
1 pair	Tweezers
1	Small flashlight with extra batteries
2	Disposable thermometers
12	Gauze pads, 3 inch x 3 inch
3	ABD/surgical pads
2	Ace bandages, 2 inch
2	Ace bandages, 4 inch
3	Kerlix rolls, 4-$1/2$ inch
3	Kling rolls, 2 inch
1	Dermicel/cloth tape, 1 inch
1	Dermicel/cloth tape, $1/2$ inch
Assorted	Adhesive bandages
1	Trauma dressing
2	Tongue depressors
2	Instant cold packs
1	Instant hot packs
1	Emergency blanket
2	"Red" bags
3	Small plastic bags
1	Bottle of eye-irrigating solution
1	Contact lens case
2	SOAP forms with pens (carbon paper if needed)
1*	Obstetrical delivery kit (optional)
***	Adrenaline ampoule with syringe (by standing orders) and small sharps container

*Items are optional on the basis of student population.

Staffing

School nurses are licensed professionals and are therefore expected to respond to emergencies in a manner similar to that of licensed nurses in other settings. In addition, practice standards have been developed by professional nursing organizations, such as NASN.

Under the best of circumstances, all schools should have on-site nursing. However, staffing levels are quite variable in schools throughout the United States. Emergency care may thus be initiated by other school personnel. Such personnel should be strongly encouraged to become certified in CPR and first aid. School nurses should take the lead in coordinating a training effort and in verifying the credentials of personnel who are assigned to respond in an emergency situation. School employees responding to emergencies should be taught to use universal precautions and have personal protective equipment available.

If a nurse is covering several school sites, he or she may need to perform telephone triage of problems that arise and advise other personnel to act accordingly. The use of telephone triage protocols may aid in the proper categorization of problems and increase the likelihood of a good patient outcome.

Linkage of School With Other Healthcare Physicians

EMS

When a school emergency arises, activation of the EMS system may be a crucial link in the chain of emergency care. The school nurse must have an understanding of the configuration of the EMS system in the community. This understanding includes knowledge of the training and expertise of responders, the planned response and arrival time of the responders, the availability of specialty transport teams and vehicles (helicopters or fixed-wing aircraft), and the existence of field treatment and destination policies and protocols. It is also important to know who is providing medical direction for the EMS services.

The name, location, and telephone numbers of the EMS system contacts should be posted in a highly visible place in both the nurse's and the administrative offices. Emergency activation through the use of the 911 system is not universal in the United

States. There are still places that use Public Service Access Points (PSAPs) with seven-digit numbers. Heightening the awareness of appropriate 911 usage by students and school staff increases the likelihood of rapid arrival by EMS when needed. Public education tools and kits, such as the "Make the Right Call" developed by the National Highway Traffic Safety Division, are useful for this purpose.

Community Emergency Departments

When care of a child has been transferred from school health personnel to EMS physicians after a school emergency, the child will be transported for definitive care to a local hospital emergency department. Schools should post the telephone numbers of the nearest hospitals and be aware of the distance and transport times. There may be circumstances when families request transport to a particular hospital or to a specialty hospital to meet the special needs of their child. Schools should have a clear policy on what to do if this situation arises and to make sure that the request is in compliance with school, EMS, and state and local policy. School health personnel can coordinate this effort and ensure good communication between all parties.

When an emergency transport to a hospital occurs, a designated person should inform parents or guardians of the EMS destination. Likewise, information must be conveyed to hospital emergency department personnel. The school nurse is the best person to convey information about the student's health status, the actual events of the emergency, and the initial on-scene assessment and management of the child's condition.

Local hospital emergency departments often have personnel interested in educating people in the community, particularly in the area of injury prevention and control. School-based health programs should take advantage of the expertise of emergency physicians and nurses and attempt to provide educational programs for students and staff. Examples of such programs are bicycle-safety demonstrations and first aid and CPR courses. Often EMS agencies are active participants in these public information efforts as well. School nurses should take the lead in coordinating these programs to strengthen health partnerships between schools, EMS, and hospitals.

Primary-Care Physicians

A crucial link in the chain of emergency care for children is the primary-care physician. Primary-care physicians not only provide well-child screening and preventive services, but also assume responsibility during and after acute illnesses and injuries and ensure that patients are referred to specialists when appropriate. They are the overall coordinators of care and must be kept abreast of any emergencies that arise. Primary-care physicians for children are often strong advocates for schools and school programs and should be seen as partners in trying to secure the best possible resources for dealing with school emergencies.

The school nurse is the best person to facilitate communication between the primary-care physician and the school. In a life-threatening situation, primary-care physicians should be immediately informed of where the child was taken for care. In other situations, communication may be delayed and can even be done by parents and caretakers. When a child returns to the school environment subsequent to an acute emergency, it is the responsibility of school health personnel to communicate with physicians to learn of any new health conditions or restrictions that the student may have. Schools should maintain documentation of contact information for the primary-care physician for each student if possible. This is especially true for CSHCN.

Many children do not have access to primary health physicians and thus do not have access to appropriate wellness and preventive care measures. Studies have shown that access to primary health services is associated with improved health status and reduced hospitalizations and emergency department use. Some schools have set up school-based health centers in response to this problem. These centers make health services available to children through nurse practitioners. Advantages of these centers include improved access to multiple primary-care services, decreased visits to emergency departments, decreased hospitalizations, and possibly decreased cost of care. In some communities, these school-based clinics are the major source of primary care for the children in the community. These clinics should be prepared to manage emergencies in a manner similar to that of the office practitioner and have links to the community emergency department and EMS system (see Chapter 8).

Children With Special Health Care Needs at School

As a result of the Individuals with Disabilities in Education Act passed by Congress in 1990, more chronically ill and technology-dependent children are attending regular schools. A study of Massachusetts school children revealed that 1 in 1000 is dependent on medical technology on a daily basis. There is little information on the preparedness of schools and school-based health programs to deal with the challenges that these children present. Even less is known about the ability of schools to respond to emergencies affecting CSHCN.

A survey of 20 school nurses in Connecticut, 4 of whom were interviewed in detail to explore their experiences in giving care to children who require medical technology, showed that most had cared for one or two students with one or more types of technology. These nurses generally felt competent in dealing with technology-dependent children with the exception of performing emergency reinsertion of a tracheostomy tube or assessing the safety of a child on a mechanical ventilator. Advanced preparation was cited as the most important factor contributing to their competence. Given the potential morbidity and mortality associated with the emergency complications of technology-dependent children, specialized training is important for school health personnel who deal with such children (see Chapter 15).

A larger study conducted in Pennsylvania determined the number and kinds of special needs of children in regular school settings, the services that they required, and the school personnel delivering the services. Most programs employed a full-time registered nurse and a part-time physician, who was often a general practitioner (69%) rather than a pediatrician (17%). The most common chronic problems encountered were asthma, seizure disorders, hyperactivity, diabetes, cardiac disabilities, and cerebral palsy. Inhalation treatments and serum glucose monitoring were at the top of the list of services being given, but other more technical procedures also were reported with considerable frequency (Table 29).

Table 29.

Reported Health Services Provided in Decreasing Order of Frequency

Inhalation therapy or treatments
Oral medications
Serum glucose monitor
Wheelchair transfer
Bladder catheterization
Brace application
Peak flow readings
Urine glucose monitoring
Intramuscular medications
Nasogastric feeds
Colostomy care
Oxygen administration
Tracheostomy care
Ileostomy care
Central venous line care
Intravenous medications
Ventilator care
Catheter irrigation
Vesicostomy tube care
Sterile suctioning

Source: Modified from Bradford BJ, Heald P, Petrie S. Health services for special needs children in Pennsylvania schools. *J Sch Health.* 1994; 64:258–260

The SNEMS-C curriculum recommends having an Individualized Emergency Medical Plan (IEMP) for all children with a chronic health disorder. An IEMP organizes the emergency care in laymen's terms and should be developed by the school nurse with a parent and primary health physician. It should be immediately available and should be used to train other staff to take appropriate actions when an emergency arises. Specifically, an IEMP includes a step-by-step action plan for each problem, a chain of command for school management of the problem and for making parental contact, and an emergency data sheet. It also includes the telephone numbers of primary-care physicians and specialists, as well as requests for transport to a particular emergency department for specialized care. This last item may require special preplanning with the local EMS system. The appropriate emergency department to which to transport CSHCN should be part of the individualized plan. Primary-care physicians are an important resource for the school system and can serve as consultants on school readiness for emergencies.

More studies are needed to determine the exact needs of CSHCN who attend regular schools. Schools that provide education to CSHCN should have adequately trained nurses on staff and a definitive chain of command established for emergencies that may arise in the absence of a nurse. Additional school nurses should be available in proportion to the CSHCN population within a school district. An integrated healthcare approach between schools, EMS, local hospitals, and medical physicians is essential to providing an optimal environment in which CSHCN can learn.

Disaster Plan

All schools must have plans for mass casualties in the event of a disaster. The plan must be integrated into that of the community and EMS agency. It should include necessary equipment and supplies, evacuation plans, transport to receiving facilities, integration with command control, and other key elements of all disaster plans (see Chapter 15).

Summary

Schools must be prepared to manage medical emergencies. The following key points are critical in the organization of an emergency plan for the school:

- Any type of emergency may occur in the school setting; therefore schools should have a comprehensive written policy for the management of all aspects of an emergency.
- All schools should have a basic emergency supplies kit.
- School personnel required to respond in an emergency should become certified CPR and first-aid physicians.
- School health personnel should be familiar with the local EMS system and develop collaborative relations with EMS physicians.

- School health personnel should maintain communication with local emergency departments, hospitals, primary-care physicians, parents, and caretakers before, during, and after emergencies.
- Schools attended by CSHCN should consider maintaining an adequate number of health personnel specially trained to deal with the particular emergencies of technology-dependent children and maintain an IEMP for such children.
- Schools should incorporate injury- and illness-prevention activities into their health curricula, drawing on the expertise of community health physicians.

Suggested Reading

Bradford BJ, Heald P, Petrie S. Health services for special needs children in Pennsylvania schools. *J Sch Health.* 1994;64:258–260

Brainerd EF, ed. *SNEMS-C School Nurse Emergency Medical Services for Children Program: School Nurse Manual.* University of Connecticut, Department of Pediatrics. Washington, DC: Department of Health and Human Services, Health Resources Services Administration, 1996

Fryer GE, Igoe JB. Functions of school nurses and health assistants in U.S. school health programs. *J Sch Health.* 1996;66:55–58

Heneghan AM, Malakoff ME. Availability of school health services for young children. *J Sch Health.* 1997;67:327–332

Igoe JB. School nursing. *Nurs Clin North Am.* 1994;29(3):443–458

Lamberg L. Preventing school violence: no easy answers. *JAMA.* 1998;280:404–407

Advocating for Emergency Care of Children

Key Points for Advocacy

1. The pediatrician is a powerful advocate for local EMS-C concerns.

2. AAP-produced speakers' kits are available for advocacy efforts.

3. Local coalitions are important means of obtaining support for advocacy concerns.

Introduction

Emergency medical systems, hospitals, and emergency departments are widely assumed to be equally capable of caring for children and adults. In fact, this assumption has been proved untrue. Experience has demonstrated that children's needs have been (and continue to be) overlooked in emergency medical care. Although progress in the past decade has been substantial, advocacy is more important than ever in EMS-C.

Advocacy and Pediatricians

Advocacy is a means of community problem solving and public policy change. Giving of one's time to a community to improve the lives of children and families is one of the finest examples of professional service and civic participation. The importance of advocacy in the practice of pediatrics is manifested in the fact that the 1997 residency training requirements include advocacy education. Long before these guidelines were established, however, pediatricians were working as leading advocates for children. The advocacy role for pediatricians is a natural extension of their practices. Pediatricians have a unique understanding of the global issues affecting children and a critical role in prevention and primary, emergency, and specialty care. In addition, the pediatrician is a respected member of the community who can provide local leadership on community-specific issues. Because pediatricians are exceedingly aware of the availability and quality of emergency services that their patients receive, they are in an ideal position to be community advocates for EMS-C.

Advocating for EMS-C

An advocate for EMS-C has many possible ways to effect improvement in care. The process is defined by both the particular EMS-C project chosen and the mechanism(s) selected for advocacy. Projects may be identified locally or nationally and may be large or small. Examples of local projects might be implementation of: 911 emergency response, pediatric out-of-hospital care protocols, pediatric equipment standards or requirements, training programs, or prevention campaigns for injuries of regional significance. Thirteen national objectives have been defined in the EMS-C Five Year Plan published by the Health Resources and Services Administration (HRSA) and the National Highway Traffic Safety Administration (NHTSA). Objectives from the Five Year Plan are included in Table 30.

Mechanisms for advocacy can include education, lobbying, service, and coalition building, singly or in combination. Participating in public education can influence the way parents, institutions, and policy makers understand and respond to concerns regarding emergency care. Education may be done through formal group presentations or in the form of letters, e-mail, faxes, or telephone calls to legislators, policy makers, or newspapers. The average member of Congress typically receives fewer than 100 letters on any one subject. That means that your letter or letter-writing campaign can potentially carry a lot of weight. Public speaking is also a wonderful means of education. The AAP has produced a speaker's kit titled "EMS-C: A Child's Life Depends on It". The speaker's kit can be used to talk to parents, businesses, and civic groups about EMS-C. Each AAP speaker's kit includes: fully scripted text, colorful slides, audience handouts, and tips for speakers. Other EMS-C-related AAP-produced speakers' kits are: "Calming the Storm of Child Abuse and Neglect;" "Childhood Injury: It's No Accident;" and "Silence the Violence." The AAP has also produced a public education fact sheet called "When Your Child Needs Emergency Medical Services," which can be placed in the office or used as a handout. A listing of other family-oriented materials pertaining to EMS-C can be found on the Family Information Web site of the National EMS-C Resource Center (http://www. ems-c.org). In a less formal but powerful way, pediatricians can provide moving and impor-

Table 30.

EMS-C Objectives

....

Include pediatric concerns in all aspects of emergency medical services development

Develop broad-based support for improving pediatric emergency medical services

Improve and expand pediatric emergency training programs for health professionals

Ensure that prehospital and interhospital pediatric transport meets children's needs

Improve hospital classification and regional system development

Ensure access to emergency medical dispatch services for all children and their families

Ensure universal access to the emergency-care system for all children and their families

Expand the availability of injury prevention, first aid, and CPR programs

Include pediatric protocols in medical direction for all EMS agencies

Integrate pediatric components into the development of all trauma systems

Ensure a coordinated approach to EMS-C

Institutionalize EMS-C within the state EMS system

Improve data collection systems, data analysis methodology, and research to describe and evaluate emergency medical care for children

Ensure a coordinated approach to EMS-C

....

tant testimony based on their professional experience. Legislators and the media are the perfect audience for these personal messages.

Although advocacy frequently starts with the individual person, it gains strength with coalition building. The federal EMS-C Program Web site is at http://www.ems-c.org. This Web site contains information about publications, including how to obtain the complimentary guide *Reaching Out: A Guide to Effective Coalition Building.* An effective strategy is to start with organizations or systems already in place. Every AAP state chapter has a Committee on Pediatric Emergency Medicine (COPEM) chair. AAP state chapters have individual Web sites, which are linked to the AAP Web site. These sites are helpful in providing rapid access to information about state government, organizations, and possible contacts. Interested and effective collaborators include nurses, especially the Emergency Nurses Association (ENA at http://www.ena.org); emergency medical technicians (EMTs); and paramedics (National Association of Emergency Medical Technicians [NAEMT] at http://www.naemt.org); parent-teacher organizations; civic organizations; church groups; firefighters; and law enforcement authorities. The ENA Web site lists state councils and gives information for contacting state council presidents. ENA has an affiliate organization called En Care, which deals with injury prevention. The Children's Defense Fund Field Office at (202) 662-3599 provides lists of advocacy groups in state or local areas.

Sources of Information and Help

The Internet Web site of the AAP is at http://www.aap.org. Consult the AAP Web site for information prepared on Using the Internet for Pediatric Advocacy in Your State and for the section on advocacy. The advocacy section contains links to campaigns and programs relevant to EMS-C (see Chapter 9).

Examples of links from the Web site to EMS-C-pertinent campaigns include: Buckle Up America, National Emergency Medical Services Week, and National Poison Prevention Week. The National Emergency Medical Services Week is cosponsored by the American College of Emergency Physicians (ACEP). Each year, ACEP produces a media campaign kit to assist healthcare professionals in promoting efforts to improve the emergency medical care available to adults and children. The tools in this kit can help plan local activities that meet the unique needs of your community and organize projects for the future. The ACEP Web site at www.acep.org also contains other valuable resource information regarding EMS-C.

Examples of AAP Web site links to EMS-C-pertinent programs include the Firearms Injury Prevention Training Project and the Medical Home Program for Children with Special Health Care Needs.

The National EMS-C Resource Center (www.ems-c.org) serves as a clearinghouse for the collection and dissemination of products for the EMS-C Program and other information. The Center can also be reached by telephone ([202] 884-4927), fax ([301] 650-8045), e-mail (info@emscnrc.com), or mail at 111 Michigan Avenue NW, Washington, DC 20010. The National and State Activities Web page at the Center's site links to individual states for activities on grants, contacts, and legislation. It also is the site for a Web page Discussion Area meant to help facilitate discussion and networking among persons interested in similar topics. Additionally, the EMS-C Web site is a good place to start for recommendations for data sources and availability of funding.

Suggested Reading

Heffernan D, ed. Be a voice for children: some basic tips on child advocacy. *CDF Reports.* Jan/Feb 1993;14:1–3

Emergency Medical Services for Children National Resource Center. *Five Year Plan: Emergency Medical Services for Children, 1995–2000.* Washington, DC: Maternal and Child Health Bureau, Health Resources and Services Administration, and National Highway Traffic Safety Administration, Department of Transportation; 1995

Lozano P, Biggs VM, Sibley BJ, Smith TM. Marcuse EK, Bergman AB. Advocacy training during pediatric residency. *Pediatrics.* 1994;94: 532–536

Part V

Transport

Transport services are essential for children who require a higher level of care. Yet, the process of transport can be a critical point of communication breakdown and risk for the child. Considerations for safe, effective transport from the office to the hospital, as well as between hospitals, are presented in this part of the book.

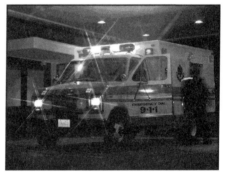

Chapter 21

Office-to-Hospital Transport

Tips for Transporting Patients From the Office

1. Have a policy and procedure in place.
2. Know your transport options and choose the one most appropriate for the patient.
3. Triage patients to appropriate receiving facilities.

Introduction

Acutely ill pediatric patients in an office setting will occasionally require referral and transfer. The receiving facilities include emergency departments, local general inpatient facilities, and local or distant pediatric inpatient units. Patients who require transport from the office can be categorized (triaged) into one of several groups: (1) stable with a nonacute medical problem, (2) moderate or potentially progressive illness, (3) urgent therapy unavailable in the office or continuation of office-initiated therapy, or (4) need for acute life-saving interventions. The potential mode (vehicle), level, and rapidity of transport depends on the patient's condition as well as available in-office treatment options and staff expertise. A well-stocked, -staffed, and -prepared office environment can offer more sophisticated diagnostic, stabilization, and interventional potential than can one less well prepared for the acutely ill patient (see Chapter 5).

Transport Options

There are several options for pediatric patient transport from the office. The first requires a nonmedical (parent, caretaker) escort to accompany the patient to the receiving facility. The mode of transport can be by car, by bus, or on foot. This method, the least-expensive transport, can be effective with a well-directed family and a patient who is not acutely ill. A potential difficulty with parental transport includes self-directed detours en route to the secondary medical location. It is not uncommon for caretakers to stop at home, pick up the other children, shop, wait for a spouse, or perform other activities prior to their planned arrival at the next facility. The parental transport may be perceived by the parent as somewhat elective because if the illness were dangerous or the child's condition were especially worrisome, the physician would have sent them in an ambulance. This opinion may be held as well by the emergency department staff. When a child arrives from a private physician's office in parental custody, that patient may be triaged as being less seriously ill or injured than one that arrives by ambulance or other mode of medical transport. If the patient is sent unaccompanied by medical personnel to another facility, notify the receiving physician and staff, not only to maintain the continuity of care, but to alert the physicians of the patient's pending arrival, to discuss the concerns of the referring physician, and to establish contact for flow of patient information. Patients who arrive at an emergency department after parental transport and for whom no contact has been made prior to transport will often be triaged with all other emergency department patients.

A second mode of nonmedical transport is by taxicab. The taxicab offers direct access to the hospital with less likelihood of interim stops. The triage issues within the hospital still apply, and there is the added confounder of potential patient safety in a taxicab. Taxicabs without functional seat belts or the ability to secure car seats for young children, as well as the unknown skills of the driver, may lead to an unsafe transport. Remember, however, that the referring physician is legally responsible for patient safety until the patient arrives at the emergency department (see Chapter 18).

Transport from the office to the hospital can be accomplished by several types of providers. A basic life support (BLS) ambulance will offer direct access to a receiving facility. Ambulance transport sends a message to the family and to the receiving center of the physician's concerns for that patient. Patients can be transported relatively safely in the belted seats or secured stretcher of a BLS ambulance. There are no specialized restraints to secure infants and children in ambulances, and state statutes vary greatly throughout the United States. A potential problem with BLS transport is the limited ability of the emergency medical technician (EMT) to offer advanced life support (ALS) should it become necessary. One advantage is that, in some systems, a parent can accompany the child in the ambulance if desired or arrange his or her own transportation to the receiving hospital. All options for transport have advantages and disadvantages. The parent who accompanies the child in an ambulance has an opportunity to direct full attention to the emotional needs of the child, rather than concentrating on driving or other matters. A major disadvantage is that the parent will be without transportation at the receiving hospital, which can be inconvenient and expensive if return transportation needs to be arranged.

Many communities rely on volunteer ambulance services. They are generally staffed by BLS providers or first responders. The positive aspects of ambulance transport, including direct access to the hospital and safety during the transport, are maintained. The volunteers, however, may have little experience in pediatric emergency care and may be certified only as first responders. If the patient may require medical intervention and no other transport services are available, the physician may need to accompany the patient in the ambulance to the receiving facility.

An ALS ambulance increases the level of potential deliverable medical care. ALS capabilities include oxygen and intravenous fluids, drugs, airway skills, and advanced support as needed. Paramedics are the ALS-level providers. The paramedic is capable of offering more sophisticated skills and expertise than does the BLS provider or first responder. Although paramedics are often skilled in ALS procedures, the amount of training and expertise in pediatric emergency care varies greatly from state to state and from emergency medical service (EMS) agency to EMS agency. It is important to remember that the paramedic is trained for extrication, critical medical intervention and stabilization, and rapid transport and is not trained for making specific diagnoses in the field.

The next level of transport is the critical care ambulance team. A critical care ambulance usually includes the addition of a critical care nurse to the paramedic-based team. This configuration has the advantages of paramedic ambulance transport with the inclusion of a skilled critical care nurse, which affords a higher level of assessment and intervention but does not necessarily include pediatric expertise. A significant potential disadvantage with the critical care ambulance team is the extrapolation of adult care to pediatric patients. Although, in many cases, this practice can be acceptable, generalizations from adult experience to pediatric care can lead to difficulties in diagnosis, intervention, and stabilization.

The most sophisticated pediatric transport is the specialized pediatric critical care transport service. These transport systems are often based at receiving pediatric hospitals, include specialized pediatric critical care transport nurses, and may include physicians at the resident, fellow, or attending level, as well as paramedics, respiratory therapists, or other medical personnel. The specialized critical care transport service affords all the aforementioned advantages as well as specialized pediatric assessment, monitoring, and perhaps diagnostic capabilities. The pediatric critical care transport service includes pediatric-specific equipment and personnel with the ability to offer critical care services in a mobile environment. Because they are often dispatched from a receiving hospital or pediatric receiving hospital, there is coordination of care between the referring hospital and the receiving institution, which can improve the efficiency of the definitive medical care. Use of the specialized pediatric critical care service allows pediatric-specific care to begin at the moment of initial patient referral and continue throughout the entire transport process. An added advantage is the availability of pediatric medical expertise at the command-physician level throughout the entire transport process. An expectation of specialized pediatric transport should be the establishment of clear avenues of communication for patient follow-up information. Telephone numbers, physician's names, and patient location at the receiving hospital should be relayed to the referring physicians, and the receiving physicians should be given contact names and telephone numbers of the referring and primary physicians. The transport service should be able to assist with patient information flow not only in the immediate transport time period, but also in the days or weeks afterward. Potential difficulties with specialized pediatric critical care services are that they are relatively expensive, are resource limited, and may not be in close proximity to the office or community hospital.

Patient Triage

ALS transport is indicated for a patient who has a life-threatening problem or has the potential to decompensate en route to the receiving facility. This transport option allows for an immediate response to the receiving facility, the ability to initiate or continue advanced life support interventions, and the ability to provide rapid transport to the facility. If necessary, a secondary transport by a specialized critical care team can be arranged when the patient has been stabilized.

Any office patient who is not undergoing an acutely life-threatening event but needs to be hospitalized in a local hospital should be transported by ambulance. If the patient is to be eventually referred to a hospital for a higher level of care that is not in the community, it is often prudent to arrange transport to a local facility for additional evaluation, intervention, and observation prior to arranging for more definitive placement. It is helpful to have this intermediate step in the transport process to allow the office to continue to function with minimal disruption. It also enables the patient to be transferred to an area where emergency care and monitoring is the norm. It allows medical studies and tests to be completed, which will help facilitate the patient's eventual admission to the receiving hospital. If the patient will eventually be transferred to a distant hospital, an intermediate transport to a local hospital may seem to be an additional, perhaps unnecessary, expense. In making those decisions, however, one must recognize and adequately assess the level of care that the child can receive in the office while waiting for transport by a specialized pediatric transport team, as well as the risk one takes in arranging for prolonged transport by a local non-pediatric-trained ambulance service.

The family, BLS ambulance, or other transport service can transport the third type of patient, one who is not acutely ill or expected to progress in severity within the transport time frame (and beyond). The primary-care physician may wish to accompany the patient being transported. However, the addition of the primary-care physician may or may not be useful, depending on the mode of transport. For example, if a patient is transported by private car, the addition of a physician does not add much to the potential intervention capabilities for that patient. It is very difficult to intervene in an automobile, especially without ALS equipment, medications, and additional personnel. Although the addition of a physician in those situations may be emotionally reassuring, a more appropriate decision would be to accompany the patient in an ambulance. The primary-care physician who accompanies the BLS ambulance can provide pediatric expertise and direction of care but must be aware that the BLS ambulance is often not well prepared for ALS procedures. It is also important to recognize that an ambulance environment is different from a hospital or office setting and that knowledge of the idiosyncrasies of ambulance transport including suction, oxygen and air delivery, stabilization, mobilization, radio, communications, motion, and environmental concerns are critical. The addition of the primary-care practitioner to an ALS ambulance can often increase the potential level of care provided to the patient. One must recognize, however, that the ALS ambulance provider has a medical direction from standardized protocols or the base hospital. The management instructions may be different from, or in conflict with, those of the primary-care physician. The physician, however, can offer pediatric expertise and guidelines that may complement the technical skills of the ALS provider. In some states, an accompanying physician may assume responsibility for patient care even if ALS providers are under medical control. Remember that these situations are generally not covered by medical liability or Good Samaritan laws. The addition of a primary-care physician to a specialized pediatric critical care ambulance is usually not necessary. A pediatric critical care ambulance service should have full pediatric capabilities and may indeed have more directed interventional capabilities than the primary-care physician may have. If the primary-care or referring physician does desire to accompany the patient in the pediatric critical care ambulance, the physician should discuss individual responsibilities during the transport with the transport personnel or medical director or both. A well-developed pediatric critical care transport service can manage and intervene for most critically ill pediatric patients and the addition of a "nonteam member" may decrease the efficiency of the participants in the team.

Another situation to be considered is the patient who requires specialized transport from the home to the office or from the office to the home. This situation is particularly relevant for children with special health care needs (CSHCN). When there is an acute emergency, the most appropriate transport service for these children is usually the local emergency medical service. EMS transport is rapid and can transfer the patient to a local facility for further assessment and stabilization. Potential difficulties with these referrals are a lack of physician assessment and participation (except by telephone) prior to the transport and the inability to further intervene or treat prior to arrival of the specialty team. If the condition of the child can be verified as nonacute and further evaluation in an emergency department is not indicated, consideration can be given to direct transport to the office, home, or other facility. However, these patients are often medically complex and may require the skills of an EMS physician and local emergency department staff. This is a situation in which the inclusion of the home healthcare professional or parent knowledgeable of the transport process is appropriate.

Preparations and Other Considerations

It is imperative that the office physician and staff be aware of options for patients who may potentially need transport. This knowledge is best acquired prior to the initiation of a transport. Be aware of the options for transport from the office in a particular location and whether they include volunteer, BLS, ALS, critical care, or specialized transport capabilities. Contact telephone numbers for the ambulance and transport services should be in a central location. Ideally, there should be contact with the ambulance service prior to the need for a particular transport so that a relationship is developed between the service and the office. As part of developing this relationship, the ambulance service may be able to visit the office and identify matters that may help in ensuring safe and efficient transport. These matters include preparation of specific directions to the physician's office and identification of parking, patient transfer locations, areas within the office from which the patient can be efficiently transported, and areas from which transport may be very difficult. The receiving hospital options should be explored prior to the need for transport and, if there are variable options, the most appropriate one should be chosen for the individual patient. Receiving hospital and physician telephone numbers and protocols for referring a patient to a hospital should be readily accessible. The office medical personnel (physicians, nurses, and other practitioners) should have up-to-date pediatric stabilization skills [cardiopulmonary resuscitation (CPR), pediatric advanced life support (PALS), and advanced pediatric life support (APLS)]. Adequate resuscitation equipment should be available in the office.

It is important to recognize that keeping a relatively ill or progressively deteriorating child in an office setting awaiting a specialized transport service can be a disservice to the patient. If there is only a potentially short delay for a pediatric critical care transport service to arrive at an office and the patient can be adequately stabilized without the need for further diagnostic tests or more sophisticated interventions, definitive transport from the office may be appropriate. However, in most situations, the patient is better off by being transferred by ALS to a community emergency department, where the patient can be observed and stabilized while waiting for the arrival of the specialized pediatric service. Most offices cannot offer the monitoring and diagnostic capabilities of the community emergency department. Keeping an ill patient in an office setting can be stressful for the physician and staff caring for the patient, as well as for other families in the office. There is the potential for nonmedical personnel to be assigned medical roles, such as observing the patient or transferring information about the patient to a referring service, both of which are inappropriate and can lead to patient compromise. The primary function of the medical transport is to ensure that patients are safely transferred to a location that provides them with an appropriate level of care. An important component of that process is the physician's transfer of information and the advice and direction offered by experienced pediatric emergency and critical care physicians. The history is best presented by the referring physician.

Concerns regarding additional cost to the patient of an initial transport to a local hospital while awaiting a pediatric critical care transport are largely unjustified. The cost of a local transport and short emergency department stay in a general hospital will likely be small compared with the total medical cost for a child who needs specialized pediatric hospitalization. The physician who maintains a child in the office to avoid potential cost to the patient has in fact shifted the cost from the ill patient's family to the physician. The physician and staff may not be available to see other patients. Prior arrangements and contingency plans for office coverage and patient rescheduling should be available for these occasions, especially if the physician chooses to accompany patients during the transfer. Although assessment of insurance status should never delay an emergency transport, it must be considered for the nonurgent patient. Transfer of a patient by a noncovered ambulance service to a noncovered institution is not in the patient's or physician's best interest. Prior knowledge of insurance limitations or preferred vendors for ambulance services and institutions in the local area can be quite useful.

Pediatricians should consider using their expertise to augment the interventional and advanced life support skills of the local out-of-hospital care personnel and perhaps even those of the general emergency department staff. This educational effort can yield significant dividends if done routinely.

When an ambulance is called to an office, clear instructions on how to get to the office, the location of a convenient and safe place to park, and the best way to access the patient-care area (back door and so forth) are mandatory. Although these instructions are not major concerns for local ambulance companies, a lack of directions can lead to significant delays for the out-of-town specialized service. There must be an entrance through which the ambulance stretcher and equipment can be easily maneuvered. Physician involvement with ambulance or critical care services promotes more efficient information flow, including direction to the office's parking areas and where the patient can be expected to be located, which can ensure a more rapid arrival of the transport service and a smoother transition of care.

When a patient is transferred from the office to a hospital, efficient flow of medical information is very important. Give an initial condensed report of the demographics and telephone number of the referring physician, acute medical history, pertinent past medical history (allergies, infectious disease exposures, previous hospitalizations, and underlying medical issues), current vital signs, physical examination, laboratory values, interventions, and the results of those interventions (Table 31). Send copies of all pertinent material (medical documentation, parental consent, and diagnostic studies, including copies of radiographs) with the transport team. Assist the transport service with transfer of the patient as necessary. Notify parents of the need for transport and obtain consent. All these measures will ensure a smooth and rapid transport.

In the rare event of rotor wing (helicopter) transport from an office setting, advanced preparation is important. The anticipation and management of details prior to transport, such as exact

---

Table 31.

Checklist for Patients Transported From the Office

1. Telephone numbers and addresses of ambulance providers along with the level of services offered by the company or agency (BLS, ALS, and so forth).
2. Telephone numbers and directions to the local community emergency department used by the practice.
3. Telephone numbers of air transport physicians in the community and the type of services provided (ie, rotary or fixed wing).
4. Telephone numbers and directions to the pediatric receiving facilities.
5. Consents for transfer.
6. Copies of the medical record.
7. Copies of all diagnostic tests, including radiographs, and the telephone number of the facility performing the tests.
8. Documentation of the name of the ambulance provider making the transport and the time at which it was made.
9. Documentation of the person accepting the transfer at the receiving hospital and the time at which it was made.
10. A transport kit, if the practice routinely sends a physician to accompany the patient. The kit should include: resuscitation drugs, airway management equipment and supplies, supplies for vascular access, and IV fluids.

location of the office and potential landing zones, are crucial. During the actual transport, coordination and cooperation with local emergency medical systems and police and fire departments are mandatory.

It is important to recognize the medical and legal implications of transport. A physician who transports a patient from the office in a private vehicle, a taxi, or a volunteer or BLS ambulance assumes complete responsibility for the care of that patient until arrival at an appropriate medical center (see Chapter 18). When an ALS, critical care, or specialized pediatric critical care service is used, the responsibility of the patient is shared between the transport service and the referring physician. Although case law regarding the transfer of these patients is limited, it is generally accepted that the primary-care physician is totally responsible for the patient until the patient has been accepted by the transport system or receiving center, at which point the liability for the patient begins to shift. At the point at which the transport service has received the patient, it accepts progressively more responsibility. By the time of arrival at the receiving center, the referring physician should be relieved of further medical liability for the patient.

Summary

It is important to anticipate cases for which transport from the office may be necessary. Triage these patients by level of medical illness, ability of the office to effectively intervene in care, and the capabilities of the planned transport service.

- Understand and be aware of transport options in your area.
- Develop relations with ambulance providers, emergency departments, and receiving hospitals.
- Have telephone numbers and preprinted directions to the office available.
- Be aware of potential advantages and disadvantages with various types of transport.
- Consider the opportunities to improve generalized services with specialized pediatric education. Train medical personnel in first aid and basic and advanced life support.

- Be prepared for emergencies with appropriate equipment, medications, personnel, and preassigned roles.

- Anticipate the potential need of transport and notify the receiving facility as early as possible to prevent potential delays in definitive patient care.

Suggested Reading

Altieri M, Bellet J, Scott H. Preparedness for pediatric emergencies encountered in the practitioner's office. *Pediatrics.* 1990;85:710–714

Baker MD, Ludwig S. Pediatric emergency transport and the private practitioner. *Pediatrics.* 1991;88:691–695

Bolte R. Responsibilities of the referring physician and hospital. In: McCloskey KAL, Orr RA, eds. *Pediatric Transport Medicine.* St. Louis, MO: Mosby; 1995:33–40

Byron LG. The rural pediatrician's perspective. In: McCloskey KAL, Orr RA, eds. *Pediatric Transport Medicine.* St. Louis, MO: Mosby; 1995: 585–591

Foltin GL, Cooper A. Prehospital transport: ground. In: McCloskey KAL, Orr RA, eds. *Pediatric Transport Medicine.* St. Louis, MO: Mosby; 1995:553–567

King B. "Interfacility" transport from the home or office. *Pediatr Emerg Care.* 1997;13:164–168

Kronick JB, Frewen TC, Kissoon N, et al. Influence of referring physicians on interventions by a pediatric and neonatal critical care transport team. *Pediatr Emerg Care.* 1996;12:73–77

Sapien R, Hodge D 3rd. Equipping and preparing the office for emergencies. *Pediatr Ann.* 1990;19:659–667

Schweich PJ, DeAngelis C, Duggan AK. Preparedness of practicing pediatricians to manage emergencies. *Pediatrics.* 1991:88:223–229

Seidel J. Preparing for pediatric emergencies. *Pediatr Rev.* 1995;16: 466–472

Tellez D, Balazs K, Young L. Prehospital transport: air medical. In: McCloskey KAL, Orr RA, eds. *Pediatric Transport Medicine.* St. Louis, MO: Mosby; 1995:568–584

Zaritsky A, French JP, Schafermeyer R, Morton D. A statewide evaluation of pediatric prehospital and hospital emergency services. *Arch Pediatr Adolesc Med.* 1994;148:76–81

Chapter 22

Interfacility Transport of Pediatric Patients

Tips for Interfacility Transport

1. Have advanced preparation.
2. Know the transport resources available.
3. Triage patients to appropriate receiving facilities.
4. Communicate with the receiving facility.
5. Obtain and document consent for transport.

Introduction

Interfacility transport has become increasingly important and complicated. Pediatric receiving hospitals have been shown to improve patient outcomes; however, at the same time, changes in reimbursement policies have compromised the ability to choose the appropriate treatment sites.

This chapter will focus on the transportation of a patient from a referring institution to a receiving hospital. For children who are not critically ill or injured, most transfers from physician offices or freestanding urgent-care centers can be adequately managed by private car or local ambulance to the nearest hospital, from which, if needed, further transport to a higher level of care can be accomplished. (See Chapter 21 for information on transport of patients from the office.)

Advance Preparation

Advance preparation by hospitals for interfacility patient transport will not only facilitate the transport process itself, but also improve patient outcomes through more efficient and safe transport to an appropriate treatment facility. All hospitals should have in place a policy and procedure for interfacility transport of pediatric patients. The procedure should include a list of pediatric receiving hospitals and their telephone numbers; a list of transport systems with pediatric capabilities; and administrative protocols, such as transfer papers, transfer agreements, consents, and so forth, that are available and ready for use. Referring hospitals should work toward the goal of having written pre-arranged contracts with pediatric receiving hospitals.

The referring hospital should investigate the pediatric capabilities of local EMS systems serving its area. An equipment and supplies pack with the appropriate pediatric equipment should be prepared for patients who may be transported by public or private providers who do not have pediatric equipment available. Staff who accompany a child on transport must know how to operate all equipment and be able to assess the critically ill or injured child.

Transport Methods

The goal of interfacility transport is the delivery of the patient to the pediatric receiving hospital in the best possible condition. After a decision has been made for secondary transport of an ill or injured child, important consideration must be given to the appropriate mode of transport and the transport team composition. The options for the types of transport include: (1) transfer by private automobile; (2) use of a local EMS service; (3) use of a local EMS service with accompanying support personnel such as a nurse, physician, or respiratory therapist from the referring hospital; (4) use of a critical care transport team transporting all ages of patients; and (5) use of a dedicated pediatric or neonatal transport team.

Choosing the appropriate method for transport can be difficult. All types of transport teams may not be available to a given region or the resources available may be limited. The rapidity of transport from the referring hospital to the pediatric receiving center is rarely more important than the level of care available during the crucial out-of-hospital transport time. The only situation in which the speed of transport is paramount is when the physical facility of the receiving hospital is needed immediately for lifesaving procedures. Waiting for an appropriate transport team is preferable to transporting a patient with personnel who cannot provide definitive care to the child. The critical care transport team provides a mobile intensive care environment, effectively bringing the intensive care unit (ICU) to the patient. Thus there is no break in the continuum of maintaining or increasing levels of care, and the patient is afforded the best chance of an optimal outcome.

Advantages of interfacility transport by private automobile include decreased cost and forgoing the use of resources and vehicles that may be needed for other, more critical patients. Disadvantages include complete loss of control over the medical care of the patient and unexpected delays, such as the parents going home to pack clothes prior to taking the child to the receiving hospital or deciding that the child is not sick enough to justify the trip at that time. Be aware that, under federal and most state statutes, the referring physician is legally responsible for the care of the child until the child's care is relinquished to the staff of the receiving facility (see Chapter 18). If the referring physician strongly believes that a higher level of pediatric care is necessary and is unsure of the family's commitment to seek that care in a timely manner, local ambulance transport may be more appropriate.

Advantages of using a local EMS ambulance service include speed of one-way transport, relatively low cost, and maintenance of some level of medical control during transport. Disadvantages of this method include lack of sophisticated equipment or appropriately trained and experienced personnel to manage a pediatric emergency and loss of local EMS resources in the community. Studies have shown that emergency medical technician (EMT) training in pediatric emergency care is often limited and that advanced life support interventions may not be possible when the standard EMT-attended ambulance transport is used. For a critically ill or injured child who has the potential for deterioration during transport, the disadvantages of a local basic EMS ambulance transport far outweigh the advantages. The addition of a nurse or physician from the referring hospital can enhance the level of care available. However, any team member (EMT, nurse) should not be expected to provide care that is not already a routine part of that person's scope of practice. If a local EMS ambulance is used for interfacility transport, the patient should be stable and should not require advanced life support (unless the providers are specifically trained in pediatric advanced life support and emergency care), and the referring physician should feel comfortable that the patient's condition will not deteriorate during transport.

Some advanced life support (ALS) units can provide sophisticated care and monitoring during transport.

Decisions regarding the configuration of the transport team will depend on the condition of the patient, the availability of the desired transport personnel, and the time needed for definitive care.

When there is a choice between an all-age transport service and a dedicated pediatric team, advance knowledge of team capabilities is necessary. Critical care transport teams are usually trained and experienced in the care of trauma and adult cardiac patients. An all-age team may have members who are also having training and experience in the care of pediatric patients or they may have minimal training and experience with only rare pediatric transports. Most teams have some pediatric experience, although all-age teams will rarely have the level of care available from a pediatric and neonatal-only team. An all-age team with minimal pediatric capabilities is not an appropriate choice if a pediatric team is available, even if the pediatric team takes longer to arrive. The exception is for the patient needing immediate care at a pediatric receiving hospital, such as emergency surgery, when time to definitive care is important. If an all-age team is used, ask the following questions before engaging its services:

- What specific pediatric training is provided to team members?
- What past pediatric experience is needed for various types of patients?
- What is the number and percentage of annual pediatric transports?

A baseline minimum standard was set in 1991 through the Commission on Accreditation of Air Medical Services (CAAMS), a voluntary accreditation organization. The name has since been changed to the Commission of Accreditation of Medical Transport Services (CAMTS). CAMTS accreditation ensures certain basic elements of pediatric training, although the minimum level is not high.

After a team has been chosen, the vehicle selection will usually be made by the transporting organization. Critical care transport teams have access to ground and air transport units, including mobile critical care ground ambulances, rotor-wing aircraft, and fixed-wing aircraft. The type of vehicle used in transport is determined by the patient's severity of illness, space, transport personnel, distance, geography, weather conditions, cost, and safety.

Ground transport has the advantages of increased space, the ability to easily stop the vehicle for clinical assessment or procedures, and decreased cost. The primary limitation is the time necessary to complete the transport, particularly over large distances or in the dense traffic of crowded urban areas.

Helicopter transport has the advantages of speed of transport of the team to the patient and of speed of delivery of the patient to the receiving facility. Disadvantages include difficulty in monitoring the patient and performing procedures during flight, high cost, and relatively frequent lack of availability due to poor weather conditions. One successful model flies the team to the patient by helicopter with return by a ground mobile ICU. This model enables the team to reach the patient quickly, maintains the helicopter's availability for other patients if stabilization time is lengthy, and allows the advantages of ground transport during the return. The primary disadvantage is greater cost because of the use of two vehicles. Third-party reimbursement in many regions may include only the vehicle in which the patient actually travels.

Fixed-wing transport is reserved for long distances usually of greater than 100 to 150 miles. Patient assessment and intervention is usually easier than in a helicopter, because there is more space and less noise. Transport may be faster but is also more expensive than both rotor-wing craft or ground transport.

Transport Triage

Severity of illness and potential for clinical deterioration during the anticipated time of transport are difficult to predict. No objective triage tool for identifying the individual patient needing the most sophisticated resources has been validated.

Current triage tools include the judgment of the referring or receiving physician; protocols developed to use the highest level of resources for certain objectively identified patients, such as all intubated or postresuscitation patients; clinical status categorization systems; and objective tools initially developed for other purposes, including Apgar score, Glasgow Coma Scale (GCS), Pediatric Trauma Score, and Predicted Risk of Mortality (PRISM) score.

Physician judgment had been used for years before the development of more objective systems. In retrospective studies, this system generally works well if the referring and receiving physicians have significant experience in making transport decisions. The referring physician must try to determine the best choice, often without access to specialized pediatric evaluation equipment and with little experience in pediatric emergency management. The increased availability of highly trained and board-certified emergency physicians will continue to raise the standard of experience and skills in referring patients to a higher level of care. The receiving physician's decision is made without being able to examine the patient or have access to every possible test result desired. In spite of the physician's having taken all necessary steps (on the basis of best judgment), the patient may experience unexpected adverse events at any time. Individual physician judgment tends to overestimate severity of illness and need for sophisticated transport. The receiving physician making a difficult transport decision must not be a resident and should be at the fellow or attending level.

Protocols based on experience with critical care transports tend to underestimate the potential for deterioration and are frequently being replaced by patient classification systems. Studies have shown that patients who have already required a high level of intervention will be likely to require more intervention during transport. For example, intubated patients who might in the past have been considered stabilized for a lower level of transport have been shown to both frequently require reintubation, necessitating the presence of personnel skilled in pediatric intubation, and to require other significant interventions.

Clinical categorization systems are the best objective tool in current use. A transport organization may use from three to six categories with multiple clinical parameters. For example, a three-category system may place patients with no oxygen requirement in category I, those with an oxygen requirement of less than 50% in category II, and those with a higher oxygen requirement in category III. Patients with no respiratory distress, with tachypnea, or with marked distress or intubation would go into category I, II, or III, respectively. Patients with normal heart rate, tachycardia alone, or signs of shock would be similarly distributed. Then the transport team composition and vehicle are determined on the basis of the highest category entered. It may be determined that a category I patient needs a local EMS ambulance, category II patients receive a two-member critical care team, and category III patients have the highest-level team. One significant benefit of the use of individual system classification categories is that they can account for local variations in geography, distances covered, referring hospital capabilities, and available teams and vehicles.

No objective scoring system has been validated for use in interfacility transport. The most frequently studied is the PRISM score for risk of mortality in pediatric receiving centers. Multicenter studies are under way to develop transport triage tools, though it is likely that any tool developed would be used to formulate local clinical classification categories. Local variabilities in transport patterns and needs always have to be considered, and no scoring system will work equally well for teams that routinely travel hundreds of miles into very rural areas and teams with primarily urban and suburban referrals.

Communication With the Receiving Hospital

Strict laws and regulations regarding interhospital transport have significantly diminished the number of cases of transferred patients arriving without warning at pediatric receiving hospitals (see Chapter 18). This is especially true for the most critically ill patients. Not uncommonly, patients still arrive by private automobile, with X-rays or laboratory work in hand, after having been discharged from a community hospital and told to "go to Children's Hospital." These patients may arrive hours or days later than the referring hospital intended. This form of patient transfer positions the referring facility for significant potential liability. Patients requiring an ambulance or a critical care transport team have their care needs well documented, and hospital-to-hospital communication is routine.

It is the responsibility of the referring physician to identify the physician at the receiving hospital and to ensure that he or she will accept care for the patient. Although, in some systems, the two physicians may not be required to have personal contact, the referring physician must always remain available to discuss the patient's condition and management. At the time of the initial call, the referring physician should have the patient's chart available to provide detailed information including vital signs, medications given, and fluids received. Nurse-to-nurse communication from referring to receiving hospital also should be encouraged. Significant changes in the patient's status prior to transfer should be reported to the receiving physician as well as to the transport team if they are not based in the receiving unit.

As part of communication, copies of all records, radiographs, and laboratory data must be sent with the patient. A telephone number should be included to call for any results pending at the time of transfer. If any culture is positive, the patient's physician at the receiving hospital should be notified immediately. Consent for transfer to another facility must be obtained from the child's caretaker prior to interfacility transport.

Consent for Transport

All transport teams at one time or another rely on implied consent for patient transport. If the parents are not available or are incapacitated in the same event, it is assumed that they would want their child to receive the best possible care in the hope of the best possible outcome. The situation that is less clear is when the patient is not in danger of loss of life or limb and is not likely to deteriorate before parents or an appropriate designated family member can be reached.

Primary care practitioners should include in anticipatory guidance a suggestion that parents leave written permission for consent for treatment by the child's caretaker(s) in the event that the parents will be inaccessible for periods of hours or days. Telephone numbers for parental notification should be included in permission paperwork. The need for written permission to seek care extends even to a child's parent if that parent is not the child's legal guardian.

Many pediatric-only teams will request the family to stay at the referring hospital until after the team has arrived. This enables the team to obtain consent directly, additional history of the current event, and past medical history as relevant. The parents may be asked to sign consent for possible surgery in the event that they will be en route for a long period of time and thus inaccessible for surgical consent or explanation of the procedure intended. When consent for surgery is obtained prior to transfer, the transport team may be witnesses but should not be realistically expected to personally obtain the consent. The surgeon should be on the telephone with the family to properly explain the procedure as well as any risk or benefits. Always document these communications in the medical record. Consent for transport should include: the name of the receiving hospital, the type of transport team delivering care, and the name of the accepting physician.

An additional benefit of having the parents at the referring hospital is that they can be given directions to the receiving hospital and unit, as well as an explanation of visiting policies and a telephone number to call to check on the child. The team should always ask when the parents plan to come. Some parents may not be able to immediately accompany their child to the receiving hospital because of travel, work, or child care arrangements. Other parents will plan to "follow the ambulance," which should be strongly discouraged. The patient's situation will only be compounded if the family is in an accident. Three useful explanations to the family are:

- The child needs his or her family safe and sound for the emotional and physical recovery ahead.
- There is nothing the parents can do by driving dangerously to change the child's medical care.
- On arrival at the receiving hospital, getting the patient stabilized will often delay the parental visit.

The transport team should know how to get in touch with the family or relatives if the parents are en route to the receiving facility.

Reimbursement

An insurance physician may designate the hospitals at which a patient may seek care. A child with an emergency should be first taken to the nearest appropriate hospital, regardless of insurance company policies. Once stabilized, the patient can be transported by appropriate means to a "designated" hospital. Unfortunately, the optimal hospital for a particular patient's condition may not be on the insurance company's physician list. It is crucial for pediatricians and parents to advocate in advance for each insurance plan to offer at least one alternative for the highest level of pediatric care available in the area. In addition, if the primary-care physician or the family feels strongly that transfer is unsafe or not in the child's best interest, every effort should be made to take proper care of the child first and deal with the payment matters later.

Laws and regulations have mandated appropriate transfer processes for children who require a higher level of care. Insurance companies and managed-care organizations will also require incentives to cover payment for interhospital transport services; currently, many do not reimburse appropriately, if at all, for interfacility transports. What is needed but not yet available is the proof that appropriate transport can actually help to control costs by limiting ICU stays, hospital days, and the often very lengthy recovery and rehabilitation phase for children with the most severe illnesses and injuries.

Posttransport Follow-Up

The receiving physician should provide either verbal or written follow-up to the referring physician. The primary-care physician needs to be kept informed about the status of the patient and what ongoing treatment is necessary. The attending physician at the receiving hospital is responsible for providing this follow-up regarding the ongoing condition and eventual outcome of the patient. This information can be provided in the form of a written discharge summary sent immediately before or after discharge. Written consent for the release of medical records is needed.

Feedback to the transport team's medical director about the performance of the transport team is an important part of follow-up. Sometimes a team will develop a reputation for unnecessary delays, inappropriate comments, or failure to include the referring hospital's medical staff in discussions. Minor situations can lead to major misunderstandings (eg, Why did they change a perfectly good endotracheal tube? Why did they pull out our IV?), even though quite reasonable explanations exist (the tube was plugged; the IV infiltrated or was a metal needle not suitable for bumpy transport). Sometimes misunderstandings will result, and the referring hospital will simply choose to use another team in the future, even if that team does not have the appropriate pediatric capabilities. If communication problems exist between the referring and receiving physician or hospital staff, contact the medical director of the transport team to discuss these problems. Misunderstandings can often be corrected by direct communication between the parties. If there is truly a problem with the team or a team member, it can be addressed by the team's medical director. Communication of any concerns, however minor, is the key to improving patient care.

Summary

It is important to prepare to anticipate the need for interfacility transport of patients from a community hospital to a higher level of care. The type of transport must be individualized to meet the needs of every patient and should be based on many factors including:

- severity of illness or injury
- resources available in the community
- insurance company preference
- distance to the receiving hospital and weather conditions

It is important to relay all pertinent information about the patient to the receiving hospital and physician and to send all records, laboratory data, and radiological studies. Include a telephone number through which the receiving hospital can get pending test results. The receiving as well as the referral physician should receive feedback on the transport process and the patient's progress.

Avoid delay in definitive care by anticipating the need for a transport and having a protocol and procedure in place.

Suggested Reading

American Academy of Pediatrics Task Force on Interhospital Transport. *Guidelines for Air and Ground Transport of Neonatal and Pediatric Patients.* Elk Grove Village, IL: American Academy of Pediatrics; 1999

Baker MD, Ludwig S. Pediatric emergency transport and the private practitioner. *Pediatrics.* 1991;88:691–695

Beddingfield FC 3rd, Garrison HG, Manning JE, Lewis RJ. Factors associated with prolongation of transport times of emergency pediatric patients requiring transfer to a tertiary care center. *Pediatr Emerg Care.* 1996;12:416–419

Britto J, Nadel S, Habibi P, Levin M. Pediatric Risk of Mortality Score underestimates the requirement for intensive care during interhospital transport. *Crit Care Med.* 1994;22:2029–2030

Edge WE, Kanter RK, Weigle CG, Walsh RF. Reduction of morbidity in interhospital transport by specialized pediatric staff. *Crit Care Med.* 1994;22:1186–1191

Graneto JW, Soglin DF. Transport and stabilization of the pediatric trauma patient. *Pediatr Clin North Am.* 1993;40:365–380

MacNab AJ. Optimal escort for interhospital transport of pediatric emergencies. *J Trauma.* 1991;31:205–207

McCloskey KA. Emergency interhospital critical care transport for children. *Curr Opin Pediatr.* 1996;8:236–238

McCloskey KA, Johnston C. Critical care interhospital transports: predictability of the need for a pediatrician. *Pediatr Emerg Care.* 1990;6:89–92

McCloskey KAL, Orr RA. *Pediatric Transport Medicine.* St. Louis, MO: Mosby-Year Book Inc.; 1995

Moront ML, Gotschall CS, Eichelberger MR. Helicopter transport of injured children: system effectiveness and triage criteria. *J Pediatr Surg.* 1996;31:1183–1188

Orr RA, Venkataraman ST, Cinoman MI, Hogue BL, Singleton CA, McCloskey KA. Pretransport Pediatric Risk of Mortality (PRISM) score underestimates the requirement for intensive care or major interventions during interhospital transport. *Crit Care Med.* 1994;22:101–107

Seidel JS. Emergency medical services and the pediatric patient: are the needs being met? II: training and equipping emergency medical services physicians for pediatric emergencies. *Pediatrics.* 1986;78:808–812

Seidel JS, Hornbein M, Yoshiyama K, Kuznets D, Finklestein JZ, St Geme JW Jr. Emergency medical services and the pediatric patient: are the needs being met? *Pediatrics.* 1984;73:769–772

Strauss RH, Rooney B. Critical care pediatrician-led aeromedical transports: physician interventions and predictiveness of outcome. *Pediatr Emerg Care.* 1993;9:270–274

Part VI

Prevention

Successful prevention eliminates the need for many acute-care and rehabilitation services. It eliminates suffering and promotes healthy life styles. Prevention is the cornerstone of pediatric practice. This part of the book highlights three areas of prevention critical to the health and well-being of children.

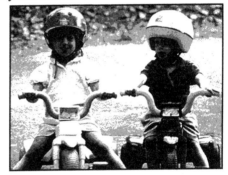

Injury Prevention and Control in a System of Pediatric Emergency Care

Key Points in Injury Prevention

1. Injury is the leading preventable health problem for children.

2. Injury prevention is an important component of EMS-C.

3. Injury prevention is an excellent area where individual involvement can make a difference. Many excellent resources are available.

Introduction

Injury prevention can be best delivered through well-integrated components of an EMS-C system. Injury prevention efforts exist at the individual, out-of-hospital, hospital, and community (city, state, and national) levels. However, all too often they are disconnected from one another. Fragmentation of efforts can result in redundancy, in creating confusion for the public and the major stakeholders, and in inefficient use of limited resources.

Models of injury prevention that have integration across disciplines and systems of care are more likely to have a positive effect, both on outcomes and on cost.

Safe Communities, described by the National Highway Traffic Safety Administration (NHTSA), is an example of a community-based model that emphasizes an integrated and comprehensive approach. It highlights the importance of interventions based on objective data, of grassroots (citizen) participation, of expanded partnerships of key stakeholders, and of evaluation of the effectiveness of programs. All components of EMS-C are included, and integration among them is critical to success.

Magnitude of the Problem

Injury is the leading preventable health problem for children. Each year, injuries claim the lives of more than 20 000 children and teenagers in the United States, which is more than all natural causes of death put together. Nonfatal injuries are responsible for more than 40% of all visits to pediatric emergency departments. Billions of dollars are spent as the result of direct and indirect expenses related to injury each year; the medical care of injured children alone amounts to $6.4 billion annually. Injury has been called the single most neglected public health problem; yet it receives a disproportionately low number of public health research dollars.

A Scientific Approach to Injury Prevention

Injury Causation

The approach to injury prevention has benefited from advances in biomechanics, behavioral sciences, and epidemiology.

The causes of injuries can be understood by investigating the host, agent (or vector), and environment interacting to create conditions that make injury likely. Whether the end result is a head injury sustained by being hit by an automobile or acute tuberculosis, it is understood that host factors (say, lack of experience in crossing the street or immunosuppression) interact with a physical environment (a busy intersection or crowded housing conditions) and an agent (the speeding motor vehicle or the tuberculosis bacterium) to create conditions that make injury or illness probable.

William Haddon, an early pioneer in injury control, built on this epidemiologic model to define his well-known "phase factor" matrix. He added another dimension to the model, that of time. Factors that contribute to the probability of the occurrence of an injury-producing event are evident in the pre-event stage; factors that influence the degree of damage to the host are evident in the event stage; and factors that mitigate the effect of the injury on the host are evident in the postevent stage. The matrix (Table 32, in which firearm injuries serve as the example) allows consideration of all the epidemiologic dimensions at each phase in time, the development of risk-factor hypotheses, and the determination of points of intervention. Typically, EMS-C with rapid emergency response belongs to the postevent stage. However, prevention activities, occurring in the pre-event stage, also are within the purview of EMS-C.

In summary, although commonly referred to as "accidents," injuries are all but random, unpredictable tragedies. Like other

Table 32.

Haddon Matrix: Application for Firearms

	Epidemiologic Dimension			
Phases	**Human Factor**	**Agent or Vehicle**	**Physical Environment**	**Socioeconomic Environment**
Pre-event	Age Experience Psychological status	Built-in safety lock	Separation of gun and child: lock box Metal detectors	Child access prevention laws
Event	Bulletproof garments	Caliber and type of bullet Automaticity		Banning of certain types of ammunition
Postevent	Age Physical condition		EMS-C systems Trauma centers	Political support for EMS-C

diseases, injuries have patterns, defined risk factors, and distinct preventive interventions.

Types of Interventions and Examples

Commonly called the "three E's," injury prevention strategies typically fall into three major groups: education, engineering (including environmental change), and law enforcement. Many of the early efforts in injury prevention included some form of *education* exclusively. Many injury-prevention education efforts remain unevaluated; many that have been evaluated have been shown to have little or no positive effect. Programs that have been effective have emphasized not only the danger inherent in certain behaviors, but also the advantages of alternative behaviors. *Engineering* changes have resulted in many lives saved in the past few decades. Despite the fact that the average American drives more miles than ever before, deaths on the roadways in the United States have fallen significantly since the early 1960s, and credit has largely been given to the physical modifications in automobiles and highways. Biomechanical advances such as seat belts and airbags have saved thousands of lives.

Enforcement of laws related to injury prevention cannot be disputed. For instance, we know that when a primary seat belt law is in place (which allows law enforcement to stop an automobile for violation of the seat belt law alone), then seat belt usage increases significantly. It is important to note that the leadership of health professionals has been key in making such legislative change happen. The first US child-safety seat law was passed in 1977 as the result of the hard work and persistence of Robert S. Sanders, a pediatrician.

The most successful approaches have been those that combine all of the "E's" of intervention. An example of such a program can be found in the Oklahoma City burn-prevention project. This successful project utilized geographic targeting with identification and intervention in the neighborhoods at highest risk of residential fires. Intervention consisted of enforcement of building codes (enforcement), reliance on smoke detectors (environment), and large-scale community awareness efforts (education). This program added an additional "E"—that of evaluation. The success of the program was measured by comparing the injuries due to residential fires in the intervention area with those in a nonintervention area.

Interventions to prevent injury may also be thought of as "active" or "passive," depending on the requirements for behavioral change in the potentially injured person or his or her caretaker. Active interventions rely on actions taken by the child or the child's caretaker (eg, storing medicines away from a child's reach or teaching the child not to touch a hot stove). The success of passive interventions, on the other hand, does not depend on efforts by the caretaker (eg, the packaging of medicines in sublethal quantities or a low temperature setting on the water heater). Most interventions have both passive and active elements. For example, a bicycle helmet will help protect against head injury, but the helmet must be worn properly in the first place. The likelihood that an intervention will be successful at preventing injury is inversely related to the amount of individual effort required.

Choosing which injuries to prevent can be difficult, because stakeholders may have a variety of interests and priorities. The Division of Injury Control of the Centers for Disease Control and

Prevention recommends that the factors considered in choosing priorities are incidence, severity, economic costs of the injuries, and the expense and likelihood of the proposed interventions. The burden that a particular type of injury imposes on society should be balanced with the economic and political feasibility of reducing that burden.

Participation of All Components of EMS-C

EMS-C is a multidisciplinary system for providing care as well as prevention activities. All components of the EMS-C system are stakeholders in childhood injury prevention and have a number of potential roles to play. Three main spheres of activity are advocacy, direct prevention activities (education as well as improving access to known effective interventions), and research (including program evaluation). Examples of these types of activities by EMS-C components are illustrated in Table 33.

Advocacy

As experts on children, emergency medical and primary-care physicians and nonphysician emergency-care providers are respected for their opinions regarding childhood trauma care and prevention. Advocacy, defined as system change, can be on many levels, whether it is the establishment of local, institutional, or office policy or the crafting or supporting of legislative change. An often overlooked form of advocacy consists in education of elected and nonelected community leaders. It is critical to gain support of such policy makers if lasting system changes are to be made (see Chapter 20).

Direct Prevention

These interventions consist of both providing direct education aimed at host or caretaker behavioral change and improving access to injury-prevention interventions such as bike helmets and smoke detectors. Every pediatrician has engaged in injury-prevention education through anticipatory guidance aimed at eliminating hazards from patient's environments. Such anticipatory guidance is assisted through available tools such as The Injury Prevention Program (TIPP) from the AAP. The education of other health professionals and groups of concerned adults has

Table 33.

Primary Injury Prevention Across the EMS-C Spectrum

	Primary-Care Physician	Prehospital EMS	Hospital
Advocacy	Establishing office policies for staff and for parents pertaining to use of child-safety seats or seat belts Education of elected and non-elected community leaders	Testifying on behalf of injury-prevention legislation Supporting the use of standardized out-of-hospital data forms	Public position by official institutional statements on injury problems Supporting and encouraging injury-prevention legislation
Direct Prevention and Education	The Injury Prevention Program (TIPP) In-office low-cost helmet sales and educational materials	Community educational outreach Participation in prevention programs (eg, bicycle rodeos, smoke-detector giveaways)	Sponsoring continuing medical education in injury prevention and car-seat programs Low-cost helmet sales Poison control center
Research and Evaluation	Patient surveys on safe behaviors	Use of prehospital databases to ascertain seat belt usage rates, etc.	Sponsor research programs or fellowships (or both) in injury prevention Utilize ICD-9 E-Codes

become easier with such resources as readymade speaker's kits available from the AAP. Speaker's kits are available on a wide range of topics including guns, EMS-C, abuse and neglect, and injury prevention in general (see the Resources section at the end of this chapter).

Research

Evaluation of the effectiveness of programs is critical to furthering and improving prevention goals. Common to all components of EMS-C and critical to injury-prevention research is the maintenance of accurate, standardized, linkable databases. The universal usage of international classification of disease ICD-9 E codes, which categorize injuries by the mechanism of the injury-producing event rather than the outcome (eg, fall down stairs versus head injury), is the first step in population-based injury-prevention research and surveillance. Information on injury data is available from the national EMS-C Web site at: http://www.emsc.org.

In 1995, the EMS-C Five Year Plan published a list of physician-specific objectives for childhood injury prevention. Table 34 lists them and includes a wide range of activities.

The Safe-Community Approach

The practical and effective application of injury-prevention interventions is the greatest challenge facing childhood injury-prevention efforts. Integrating the efforts of all taking part in the injury-prevention process is key to success. All components of the EMS must participate in an integrated manner to be effective. The Safe Communities approach developed by the NHTSA is an excellent example of practical application of integrated injury-prevention methods that are applicable to EMS-C. The main components of this approach are: interventions based on objective data, citizen participation, a comprehensive approach, expanded partnerships, and evaluation for effectiveness of outcomes. For further information and examples of this approach, the reader is referred to the Safe Communities Web site listed in the Resources section at the end of this chapter.

Table 34.

EMS-C Injury-Prevention Objectives by Practice Emphasis

••

1. Ensure that all communities have access to a comprehensive poison control center.
2. Increase the number and effectiveness of injury-prevention programs for children and adolescents by using state epidemiology data and proved countermeasures.
3. Increase the number of states that include injury-prevention content in all levels of EMT primary and continuing education programs.
4. Provide health professionals with greater access to continuing education in injury prevention and to materials for public presentations on childhood injury prevention.
5. Increase the number of states that encourage teachers to be trained in first aid, CPR, and injury prevention.
6. Increase the number of primary-care physicians who teach patients about child and adolescent injury prevention.
7. Increase the number of states with unintentional and intentional injury-prevention programs for children with special healthcare needs.
8. Increase the number of emergency departments using injury follow-up guidelines to reduce risk-taking behavior of children, adolescents, and their families.
9. Increase the number of third-party payers that require E-coding for reimbursement in both inpatient and emergency department settings.

••

Source: Emergency Medical Services for Children National Resource Center. *Five Year Plan: Emergency Medical Services for Children, 1995–2000.* Washington, DC: Maternal and Child Health Bureau, Health Resources and Services Administration, and National Highway Traffic Safety Administration, Department of Transportation; 1995.

Summary

Prevention is a key component of EMS-C. It is one of the best, most effective ways for the individual physician to take part in EMS-C activities. Many program-specific resources have been developed along with sources of data to use in community programs (see the Resources section at the end of this chapter). Other health professionals in the community such as EMTs/paramedics and nurses are also effective public educators in injury prevention.

Suggested Reading

Baker SP, O'Neill B, Ginsburg MJ, Li G. *The Injury Fact Book.* 2nd ed. New York, NY: Oxford University Press; 1992

National Committee for Injury Prevention and Control. Injury prevention: meeting the challenge. *Am J Prev Med.* 1989;5(suppl 3):1–303

Robertson LS. *Injury Epidemiology.* New York, NY: Oxford University Press; 1992

Wilson MH, Baker SP, Teret SP, Shock S, Garbarino J. *Saving Children: A Guide to Injury Prevention.* New York, NY: Oxford University Press; 1991

Resources

Coalitions, General Information and Funding Opportunities (with Web sites)

American Academy of Pediatrics (AAP)
http://www.aap.org
Ordering information on speaker's kits related to injury prevention (look under "research and advocacy" publications), model legislation, and a large selection of injury-prevention policy statements.

Consumer Product Safety Commission (CPSC)
http://www.cpsc.gov
An independent federal regulatory agency, this commission helps keep American families safe by reducing the risk of injury or death from consumer products. This Web site contains a wealth of information on consumer product-related dangers and injuries.

Emergency Medical Services for Children (EMS-C)
http://www.ems-c.org
An organization designed to reduce child and youth disability and death due to severe illness and injury through well-integrated acute care and prevention. Resources include fact sheets and health and safety guides.

Provides information about EMS-C priorities, current project summaries, and funding information for EMS-C projects.

Emergency Nurses Care, Inc. (EN CARE)
http://www.ena.org/encare/
An injury-prevention affiliate of the Emergency Nurses Association (ENA). Its mission is to reduce preventable injuries and deaths by educating the public to increase awareness and promote healthy life styles.

Injury Control Resource Information Network (ICRIN)
http://www.injurycontrol.com/icrin/
An excellent electronic clearinghouse for injury-prevention data and information. A dynamic list of key resources related to injury prevention and control; includes hyperlinks to major injury-prevention and research centers, national and state organizations, and many advocacy and resource centers.

Injury Free Coalition for Kids
http://www.injuryfree.org
This home page has links to several community-based initiatives throughout the United States. All programs were developed from a model based at the Harlem Hospital.

International Society for Child and Adolescent Injury Prevention
http://www.iscaip.org/
This society is a collaborative effort of childhood injury-prevention experts throughout the world. On-line access to a bulletin board and information about the journal *Injury Prevention* are helpful.

National Safe Kids http://www.safekids.com
A coalition of numerous groups participating in childhood safety throughout the United States.

Safe Communities (National Highway Traffic Safety Administration)
http://www.nhtsa.dot.gov/safecommunities/scanua/resources.html
A compendium of innovative state and community traffic safety programs. The clearinghouse acts as a dissemination point and source of information, ideas, and materials related to safe communities for those interested in a community-based approach to injury prevention.

Chapter 24

Immunization

Introduction

Prevention is an integral part of EMS-C, and effective immunization is a cornerstone of illness prevention. The purpose of this chapter is to describe the role of emergency departments in the immunization of children at risk for vaccine-preventable diseases. The scope of the chapter is limited to the rationale and strategy of the emergency department's potential role in vaccinating children—technical information on vaccination, such as tetanus prophylaxis in routine wound management, should be obtained from the AAP *Report of the Committee on Infectious Diseases (The Red Book)*.

The organization of the chapter is as follows: (1) the role of the emergency department in the immunization delivery system, (2) summary of evidence from emergency department vaccination studies and challenges to implementing emergency department vaccination programs, (3) potential program models, (4) a summary of key points, and (5) a suggested reading list.

Key Points in Immunization

1. Emergency department patients are more likely to be underimmunized than is the average child in the community.

2. Interventions that include vaccinating children in the emergency department have been very difficult to implement owing to difficulties in identifying vaccine-eligible children and to the reluctance of parents to have their children vaccinated in the emergency department.

3. Immunizing children in the emergency department has not been shown to improve immunization coverage levels substantially, and, when it has, the effect has been dampened within a few months.

continued

Role of the Emergency Department

Ideally, every child would receive routine vaccinations from his or her primary-care physician, who would practice according to the Standards of Pediatric Immunization Practices. However, the

Key Points in Immunization *(continued)*

4. Passive referral of children to physicians for immunization has not been shown to be effective at raising immunization coverage levels.

5. Interventions that have referred children to physicians for immunization using an outreach and tracking protocol have been successful at improving immunization coverage levels.

6. Children needing referral physicians include those who have no physician and those who are determined to not be up-to-date by a hand-held immunization record.

7. In outbreak situations, specific guidance for emergency department-based interventions should be determined in collaboration with the local health department.

ideal has not yet been achieved in the United States, and approximately a fifth of 2-year-old children are in need of at least one vaccination.

The emergency department has long been recognized as having special potential to reduce vaccine- preventable disease by participating in vaccination programs. Risk factors for underimmunization are similar to risk factors for emergency department utilization, and empirical evidence shows that emergency department patients are more likely to be underimmunized than are children in the community at large. Indeed, during the measles epidemic of 1989 to 1991, emergency departments were actually shown to be important sites of measles transmission. Furthermore, because it is safe to vaccinate injured children and children with mild illnesses, even if febrile, the potential effect of emergency department vaccination programs has been determined to be substantial.

The potential roles for emergency departments in childhood vaccination include:

- use of the emergency department as a vaccinating site during an outbreak of a vaccine-preventable disease such as measles

- providing routine vaccinations for children with no access to an immunization physician

- providing routine vaccinations to all vaccine-eligible children

- providing referrals to immunization physicians for underimmunized children

Two separate published recommendations describe the role of emergency departments for vaccinating children. The first is the Standards of Pediatric Immunization Practices, which recommends that all physician encounters, including emergency department encounters, should be used as opportunities for vaccinating children. The second is that of the American College of Emergency Physicians (ACEP), which also recommends vaccinating children in the emergency department.

Evidence From Emergency Department Immunization Evaluations

Several types of emergency department-based immunization programs have been tried and evaluated. A successful model implemented in Cincinnati includes assessment of emergency department patients' immunization status and referral of under-immunized children to an immunization outreach team that tracks the children's immunization status. In this program, patients were not vaccinated while in the emergency department; rather, they were referred to services. Evaluation revealed that a key element of the program was the immunization outreach team, which tracked the children to make sure that they were vaccinated. The immunization coverage level of children referred to the outreach team was 28 percentage points higher than that of children simply referred to a physician without an outreach and tracking protocol.

Programs designed to vaccinate underimmunized children in emergency departments, however, have been much less successful. Several unanswered challenges have impeded these emergency department vaccination programs. The first challenge has been to determine vaccination status. Generally, few parents have their child's hand-held vaccination record with them when visiting an emergency department. Without the hand-held record, immunization status cannot be assessed, owing to the inaccuracy of parental recall of vaccinations received. Several studies have tried unsuccessfully to create decision rules to determine vaccination status on the basis of parental recall. Calling the primary-care physician to determine the immunization status of an emergency department patient has limited effectiveness because the majority of children's emergency department visits are not during office hours.

The second challenge has been to convince parents of vaccine-eligible children to accept vaccination from a physician who is not the child's usual physician. Because reasons for emergency department visits are almost always curative rather than preventive, immunization is almost never the focus of an emergency department visit. Evidence supports the reluctance of parental acceptance as a problem. During the measles resurgence from 1989 to 1991, two Chicago emergency departments were used as vaccination sites. However, only about 40% of vaccine-eligible emergency department patients who were offered vaccination accepted it in the emergency department. In Milwaukee, only one-quarter of vaccine-eligible emergency department patients were vaccinated in the emergency department. In New York City emergency departments, less than a fifth of the eligible population was vaccinated.

Studies that have measured the effect of emergency department vaccination have shown disappointingly low effects on actual vaccination rates. A randomized controlled trial in Rochester, NY, showed an 8% increase in vaccination coverage compared with the control group, but the difference was not measurable after a few months. Similar results were found in a prospective cohort study in two emergency departments that serve low-income, high-risk populations in New York City.

Studies that have passively referred underimmunized children back to their primary-care physician, with or without a letter to the physician, have also had no measurable effect on vaccination coverage levels.

Challenges to immunizing children in the emergency department are shown in Table 35.

Potential Program Models

Given the difficulties of vaccinating children in the emergency department, what should be the role of the pediatric emergency department in childhood immunizations? One key factor is the purpose of the emergency department program. If the purpose is to control an outbreak, the role of the emergency department should be coordinated with the local health department authorities. For example, in an outbreak, the emergency department

Table 35.

Challenges to Immunizing Children in the Emergency Department

1. Determining the child's immunization status
2. Convincing the parents to permit immunizations
3. Storing and handling vaccines
4. Recording information required by the National Childhood Vaccine Injury Compensation Act in the medical record
5. Informing the primary-care physician that a vaccination was administered
6. Providing the vaccine information sheets
7. Following vaccinated children for adverse events
8. Tracking children who are behind in immunization

might be best used as a vaccinating site, especially if it serves a high-risk, undervaccinated population. However, in the current situation of low incidence rates of vaccine-preventable diseases, it is unlikely that the emergency department will be needed for outbreak control. The most appropriate role for a pediatric emergency department in the nonoutbreak situation is to identify children who are potentially underimmunized and to refer them to an physician for immunization with the capability of providing outreach and tracking. The failure of programs that provide passive referral to a physician for immunization underscores the importance of the outreach and tracking aspects of a program. The outreach and tracking program can determine true vaccination status after the emergency department visit and can ensure that referred children are seen by an immunization physician. In a collaborative model, the role of the local medical practice environment is, therefore, critical to the success of an emergency department immunization program.

Finally, well-intentioned programs may not succeed because of the failure to evaluate them critically. As part of a quality-improvement process, an emergency department immunization program should have some process and outcome measures to determine whether it is meeting its objectives. For example, if a program is set up to refer underimmunized children, one would want to find out the results of the referrals. Were the children linked with primary care physicians? Were they adequately vaccinated? A set of evaluation questions and an evaluation plan should be developed and implemented.

Summary

The emergency department plays an important role in the immunization of children during disease outbreaks. In other situations of routine immunization, the role of the emergency department is undergoing examination and definition. It is clear that children who present to the emergency department for care are more likely to be underimmunized. Yet there are many barriers to overcome to provide rapid identification and timely immunization of these children. Accessibility of records is one barrier, and parental education regarding the safety and effectiveness is another. Passive referral to primary-care physicians does not appear to be effective, and even emergency department immunization programs have been shown to have minimal long-term effect. Substantial outreach and tracking appear to be a successful means of improving childhood immunization rates. Thus support for the development of statewide and even national immunization registries that are readily available to healthcare physicians is an important priority in continuing to eliminate barriers and to increase access to immunizations.

Suggested Reading

Ad Hoc Working Group for the Development of Standards for Pediatric Immunization Practices. Standards for pediatric immunization practices. *JAMA.* 1993;269:1817–1822

Bell L. Providing primary care to children in the emergency department: a problem or a missed opportunity? *Pediatr Emerg Care.* 1991;7:124

Bell LM, Lopez NI, Pinto-Martin J, Casey R, Gill FM. Potential impact of linking an emergency department and hospital-affiliated clinics to immunize preschool-age children. *Pediatrics.* 1994;93:99–103

Farizo KM, Stehr-Green PA, Simpson DM, Markowitz LE. Pediatric emergency room visits: a risk factor for acquiring measles. *Pediatrics.* 1991;87:74–79

Goldstein KP, Kviz FJ, Daum RS. Accuracy of immunization histories provided by adults accompanying preschool children to a pediatric emergency department. *JAMA.* 1993;270:2190–2194

Humiston SG, Rodewald LE, Szilagyi PG, et al. Decision rules predicting vaccination status of preschool-age emergency department patients. *J Pediatr.* 1993;123:887–892

Joffe MD, Luberti A. Effect of emergency department immunization on compliance with primary care. *Pediatr Emerg Care.* 1994;10:317–319

Lindegren ML, Atkinson WL, Farizo KM, Stehr-Green PA. Measles vaccination in pediatric emergency departments during a measles outbreak. *JAMA.* 1993;270:2185–2189

Robinson PF, Gausche M, Gerardi MJ, et al. Immunization of the pediatric patient in the emergency department. *Ann Emerg Med.* 1996;28:334–341

Rodewald LE, Szilagyi PG, Humiston SG, et al. Effect of emergency department immunizations on immunization rates and subsequent primary care visits. *Arch Pediatr Adolesc Med.* 1996;150:1271–1276

Rodewald LE, Szilagyi PG, Humiston SG, et al. Is an emergency department visit a marker for undervaccination and missed vaccination opportunities among children who have access to primary care? *Pediatrics.* 1993;91:605–611

Schlenker TL, Risk I, Harris H. Emergency department vaccination of preschool-age children during a measles outbreak. *Ann Emerg Med.* 1995;26:320–323

Schubert C, Gay E, Wong H, Auer K, Johnston K, Meyer M. Vaccinating high risk preschoolers: linking the community with the emergency department [abstract]. *Ambulatory Child Health.* 1997;3(suppl):169. Abstract 153

Family Violence and EMS-C

**Key Points in the Identi-
fication and Treatment
of Family Violence**

1. Family violence is common.
2. Abused children frequently have mothers who are abused.
3. Screening is important to identification and intervention.
4. Safety concerns are important for the abused woman who seeks to leave the relationship.

Introduction

Family violence is the intentional intimidation, physical or sexual abuse or both, or battering of children, adults, or elders by a family member, intimate partner, or caretaker. It is common, affecting about one in four American households. Children are affected as victims, witnesses to violence, perpetrators, and future parents. Children victimized by family violence frequently access emergency services. Child abuse accounts for about 10% of the injuries to children under the age of 7 years who are examined. Thus, family violence is an EMS-C concern. This concern is clearly affirmed in the objectives of the Five Year Plan for EMS-C published by the Health Resources and Services Administration (HRSA). Battered children challenge all linkages in the EMS system from out-of-hospital care through rehabilitation. To be comprehensive and contribute to breaking the cycle of violence, a seamless EMS-C system must go beyond the victimized child and address family violence and primary prevention of all forms of abuse.

Breaking the Cycle of Violence

The recognition and management of the battered child have been well defined and are integral parts of the practice of pediatrics. Yet, when only the abused child is recognized, a very important part of the cycle of violence is neglected. Abused children frequently have abused mothers. Estimates are that their male partners physically abuse 2 million women each year. In emergency department surveys, from 2% to 4% of women report acute episodes of abuse, and lifetime incidence of violence ranges between 11% and 54%. Staff may detect as little as 5% of battered women presenting to the emergency department. Recognition of the battered woman is an important concern not only for the emergency department, but also for clinics and offices where abused mothers may bring their children for care. Abused mothers frequently have abused children. Therefore recognition begins the process of intervention. And intervention on behalf of battered women and their children may be one of the most effective means of preventing child abuse. Yet, as important as the process of recognition and intervention for the battered mother is, these are sensitive, private, and difficult situations for which the role of the pediatrician is gradually being defined. A very important step for the pediatrician is the process of personal and professional education about family violence. This education includes the dynamics of abusive relationships and the steps for managing these situations in a safe and sensitive manner. The Committee on Child Abuse and Neglect of the AAP has published a statement on the Role of the Pediatrician in Recognizing and Intervening on Behalf of Abused Women. This statement provides practical guidance and recommendations for approaches when the circumstance of family and intimate-partner violence is identified (see Table 36). A woman is at greatest risk when planning to leave an abusive relationship. Table 37 details safety concerns that can be used for counseling.

Breaking the cycle of violence in the United States is contingent not only on comprehensive medical care for victims, but also on primary prevention. It requires a multidisciplinary effort in which the pediatrician plays a critical role by participating in screening and identifying high-risk families, implementing and supporting home visitation programs, conducting parenting classes, and providing anticipatory guidance on matters such as discipline. Important risk factors have been identified for intimate-partner abuse occurring within the past year. These risk factors include:

- Age, 18–39 years
- Monthly income less than $1000
- Children younger than 18 years living in the home
- Ending a relationship within the past year

Table 36.

Pediatrician's Role in Recognizing and Intervening on Behalf of Abused Women

1. Residency training programs and continuing medical education (CME) program leaders incorporate education on family and intimate-partner violence and its implications for child health into the curricula of pediatricians and pediatric emergency department physicians.
2. Pediatricians should attempt to recognize evidence of family or intimate-partner violence in the office setting.
3. Pediatricians should intervene in a sensitive and skillful manner that maximizes the safety of women and children victims.
4. Pediatricians should support local and national multidisciplinary efforts to recognize, treat, and prevent family and intimate-partner violence.

Source: American Academy of Pediatrics Committee on Child Abuse and Neglect. The role of the pediatrician in recognizing and intervening on behalf of abused women. *Pediatrics.* 1998;101:1091–1092.

Table 37.

Safety Concerns for the Victim of Intimate-Partner Abuse

- Call a shelter. Find out about your legal options and resources available.
- Have an emergency bag prepared in a safe, confidential place. Include: clothing, cash and checks, identification, important papers, and so forth.
- Know where you would go and how to get there in the middle of the night. Keep your purse and car keys ready.
- Develop a code word to use with friends for help.
- Teach children how to call for help.

In addition to the screening of families, written materials, brochures, and posters on family violence can be displayed and placed throughout the office or emergency department and in areas such as the lavatory, where the mother will have private, unobserved access to the information.

Summary

Family violence is a pervasive problem that affects millions of children. Identification and intervention in family violence through programs in which primary-care physicians participate is important in curbing this epidemic. The cycle of abuse can be broken with appropriate intervention.

Suggested Reading

American Academy of Pediatrics Committee on Child Abuse and Neglect. The role of the pediatrician in recognizing and intervening on behalf of abused women. *Pediatrics.* 1998;101:1091–1092

Dearwater SR, Coben JH, Campbell JC, et al. Prevalence of intimate partner abuse in women treated at community hospital emergency departments. *JAMA.* 1998;280:433–438

Educating the nation's physicians about family violence and abuse. *Acad Med.* 1997;72(suppl):S3–S115

Knapp JF, Dowd MD. Family violence: implications for the pediatrician. *Pediatr Rev.* 1998;19:316–321

Resources

A national toll-free hotline is available to all physicians and victims needing information about local resources on domestic violence: (800) 799-SAFE [(800) 799-7233]. The Family Violence Web site at www.famvi.com contains a list of state toll-free hot lines, myths and facts, statistics, and personal communications and essays. Many other Web sites on family violence are listed.

American Bar Association Commission of Domestic Violence at http://www.abanet.org/domviol/home.html

Battered Women and Their Children at http://www.columbia.edu/ ~ rhm5

Domestic Violence: A Practical Approach for Clinicians at http://www.sfms.org/domestic.html

Domestic Violence Information Center at http://www.feminist.org/other/dv

Domestic Violence Shelters at http://www.zip.com.au/ ~ korman/dv/

Electronic Journal of Intimate Violence at http://alpha.acast.nova.edu/ health/psy/file-desc/file50.html

Family Peace Project at http://www.family.mcw.edu/ ahec/ed/med-viol.html

Family Violence Prevention Fund at http://www.fvpf.org

Justice Information Center at http://www.ncjrs.org/victdv.htm

Minnesota Center Against Violence at http://www.umn.edu/mincava

Shattered Love Broken Lives Domestic Violence Main Menu at http://www.st.com/projects/DomVio/

Stop Abuse for Everyone (SAFE) at http://www.dgp.utoronto.ca/-jade/safe

US Department of Justice at http:www.usdoj.gov/vawo

Part VII

EMS-C at the National Level

The Maternal and Child Health Bureau (MCHB, HRSA) of the US Department of Health and Human Services administers a federal program for the development and implementation of EMS-C throughout the 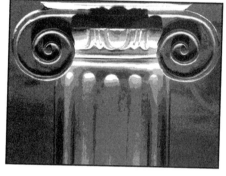 United States. This program has provided funding in many ways for EMS-C activities. This part of the book describes the federal EMS-C program.

The Federal EMS-C Program

Key Facts About the Federal EMS-C Program

1. Administered by HRSA, MCHB, and NHTSA.
2. Funds grants to states and medical schools.
3. Has funded projects in all states and many territories.
4. Provides a means for collaboration among groups concerned with pediatric emergency care.

Introduction

The federal Emergency Medical Services for Children (EMS-C) program is designed to ensure state-of-the-art emergency medical care for the ill or injured child and adolescent through grants to states and medical schools. It builds on existing EMS systems, which initially focused on adult emergency care with little attention paid to the special needs of children. EMS-C addresses the entire continuum of pediatric emergency services, from injury prevention and EMS access through out-of-hospital and emergency department care, intensive care, rehabilitation, and reintegration into the community, while ensuring the ongoing involvement of the child's primary-care physician.

The EMS-C grant program is a joint program of the Health Resources and Services Administration's (HRSA) Maternal and Child Health Bureau (MCHB) and the National Highway Traffic Safety Administration (NHTSA).

History

The groundwork for change in EMS-C was laid in the late 1970s when Calvin Sia, MD, a pediatrician and president of the Hawaii Medical Association, urged members of the American Academy of Pediatrics (AAP) to develop multifaceted EMS programs that would decrease morbidity and death in children. Dr Sia worked with Senator Daniel Inouye of Hawaii and his assistant, Patrick DeLeon, PhD, to write legislation for an initiative on emergency medical services for children.

In 1983, a particular incident served to personalize the need for these services. One of Senator Inouye's senior staff members had an infant daughter who became critically ill. Her treatment demonstrated the average emergency department's shortcomings when facing a child in crisis. A year later, Senators Orrin Hatch (Utah) and Lowell Weicker (Connecticut), backed by staff members with disturbing experiences of their own, joined Senator Inouye in sponsoring the first EMS-C legislation. Thus, the federal EMS-C program was established in 1984.

Alabama, California, New York, and Oregon became the first recipients of federal grant money specifically earmarked to improve pediatric emergency medical services. The first states, exploring innovative strategies and developing new models of care, launched an ongoing series of improvements to the EMS system. As of 1998, EMS-C grants had helped all 50 states, the District of Columbia, Puerto Rico, and three territories in making good progress toward optimal emergency care for all children.

The federal program was heavily influenced by the work of several pediatricians. For example, research by James Seidel, MD, of Harbor-UCLA Medical Center showed that outcomes for critically ill and injured children improved when children were cared for in specialized pediatric centers. He also determined that many EMS physicians did not have the training or equipment to care for pediatric patients. At the same time, Dr Max Ramenofsky's study of pediatric trauma deaths showed that errors in care resulted in an increased mortality rate for pediatric patients. These studies spurred the development of the Emergency Department Approved for Pediatrics-Pediatric Critical Care Center (EDAP-PCCC) system in the County of Los Angeles—a model subsequently used by many states to improve pediatric emergency care in EMS systems.

Modestly funded since its initial authorization in 1984, the federal EMS-C program has provided grants to states to address all of the concerns related specifically to children who experience an emergency illness or trauma. In addition, the program has increased our knowledge of how to treat children in emergency situations and has provided materials for educational programs and systems development that can be used by states in the absence of special grant funds. Despite this progress, a 1993 study by the National Academy of Science's Institute of Medicine (IOM) documented many remaining gaps and deficiencies in pediatric emergency medical services.

Institute of Medicine Report and the Five Year Plan

The IOM report included a number of recommendations designed to improve children's care in emergencies. Staff from MCHB and NHTSA joined with a panel of expert advisers, representing the spectrum of care on the EMS-C continuum, to convert the IOM's recommendations into action. The resultant draft plan was sent to individual professionals, groups, and organizations throughout the United States for review and discussion. The comments received were analyzed and integrated into a Five Year Plan for EMS-C, published in 1995.

Three years into the plan, the program had accomplished many of the proposed activities. In addition, baseline data for almost all the objectives had been collected. The availability of the data made it possible to revise the objectives and restate them in a way that is measurable. These data also provide a snapshot of the unmet needs related to pediatric emergency care, information that was not formerly available. Thus, a new document, EMS-C Five Year Plan, Midcourse Review, 1995–2000, updates the 1995 document in important ways. The Midcourse Review is an excellent resource that enables the nation to refocus attention on those areas that are most problematic. Table 38 provides an overview of the plan, including the baseline data.

Table 38.

Overview of EMS-C Five Year Plan, Midcourse Review, 1995–2000 and Baseline Data

Goal	Objectives	Baseline
A. Include pediatric issues in all aspects of EMS development	1. Increase by 20 the number of states with EMS system plans and associated regulations that address pediatric issues.	12 states
	2. Increase to 100% the number of communities that have access to a comprehensive poison-control center.	58%
	3. Increase to 50 the number of states having injury-prevention programs for children and adolescents.	44 states
	4. Increase to 40 the number of states with community-based linkages between children with special health care needs (CSHCN) programs and EMS-C programs.	27 states
B. Develop broad-based support for improving pediatric EMS	1. Increase by 10% the number of professional, voluntary, industrial, consumer, and advocacy groups participating in state EMS-C system projects.	482 groups
	2. Increase by 10% the number of national child health interest groups that serve as prominent advocates for pediatric emergency care.	39 groups
	3. Convene a national congress on EMS-C issues and encourage all interested groups to attend.	March 1998
	4. Increase by 10 the number of states that promote national public awareness of pediatric emergency medical services issues.	33 states

continued

Table 38. (continued)

Goal	Objectives	Baseline
C. Improve and expand pediatric emergency training programs for health professionals	1. Define and incorporate minimum course objectives in pediatric emergency care for dispatcher training programs.	18 topics
	2. Define essential topics in pediatric emergency care for EMT training and incorporate into EMT training curricula.	EMT-B: one essential topic
	3. Increase by 10 the number of states that require training in pediatric emergency care as a condition of EMT recertification at all skill levels.	0 states
	4. Increase by 15 the number of states that include injury-prevention content both in primary education and in continuing education programs for EMTs.	4 states 1 US territory
	5. Define minimum course objectives in pediatric emergency care for nurses, and incorporate this material into undergraduate and graduate nursing school curricula.	10% undergraduate 0% graduate
	6. Increase to 100% the number of residency programs that include training in pediatric emergency care.	Emergency medicine: 97%
	7. Increase by 10 the number of states that offer continuing education courses in pediatric emergency care and injury prevention for practicing emergency health professionals.	APLS: 27 states PALS: 50 states

continued

Table 38. *(continued)*

Goal	Objectives	Baseline
	8. Provide health professionals with greater access to materials on childhood injury prevention.	Resource directory 6 states
	9. Increase by 50% the number of states with approved continuing education programs on emergency care of technology-assisted children for EMS physicians.	
	10. Increase by 20% the number of sessions on EMS-C issues presented at national meetings of professional health and medical organizations.	19 sessions (APHA, 1996)
	11. Increase by 25% the number of EMS-C issues presented in schools of public health each year.	Injury prevention: 21 schools EMS content: 12 schools
D. Ensure that prehospital and interhospital pediatric transport meet children's needs	1. Increase to 50 the number of states and US territories that require all EMS-C recommended pediatric equipment on ambulances.	2 states (BLS) 5 states (ALS)
	2. Increase to 85% the number of hospitals that have interfacility transfer agreements for critically ill and injured pediatric patients.	36%

continued

Table 38. *(continued)*

Goal	Objectives	Baseline
E. Develop broad-based support for improving pediatric EMS	1. Increase by 50% the number of states that have adopted and disseminated pediatric guidelines for acute-care facility identification.	11 states
	2. Increase to 85% the number of hospital emergency departments that have all necessary equipment for the stabilization of ill and injured children.	46%
	3. Increase to 30% the number of rural and family healthcare physicians whose offices maintain a minimum complement of pediatric emergency equipment and supplies.	10%
F. Ensure access to emergency medical dispatch services for all children and their families	1. Increase to 8 the number of pediatric-specific protocol cards for emergency medical dispatchers (EMD).	4 protocol cards
G. Ensure universal access to the emergency care system for all children and their families	1. Increase to 30 the number of states that provide public education concerning appropriate use of 911 services.	21 states
	2. Increase by 6 the number of states with an enhanced (E) 911 system.	13 states

continued

Table 38. *(continued)*

Goal	Objectives	Baseline
	3. Increase the availability of information that will assist primary-care physicians, community health centers (CHCs), and managed-care organizations in providing guidance about the availability, location, and appropriate use of emergency services.	Baseline to be established
H. Expand the availability of injury-prevention, first-aid, and CPR programs	1. Increase by 20% the number of states that require training in both first aid and CPR for all licensed child-care physicians.	First aid: 42 states, CPR: 25 states Both first aid and CPR: unknown
	2. Increase to 10 the number of states that encourage teachers to be trained in first aid, CPR, and injury prevention.	1 state
	3. Increase by 25% the number of school districts that require proficiency in first aid and CPR as a condition of high school graduation.	14 states
	4. Increase by 25% the number of primary-care physicians who teach patients about child and adolescent injury prevention.	4000 physicians

continued

Table 38. *(continued)*

Goal	Objectives	Baseline
	5. Increase to 25 the number of states with programs for prevention of unintentional and intentional injuries in CSHCN.	15 states
I. Include pediatric protocols in medical direction for all EMS agencies	1. Increase to 30 the number of state EMS agencies that have pediatric protocols for both on-line and off-line medical direction.	18 states
	2. Increase to 30 the number of states having guidelines for interfacility transport of pediatric patients.	6 states
	3. Increase to 60% the number of emergency departments using injury follow-up guidelines to reduce risk-taking behavior of children, adolescents, and families.	53%
	4. Increase to 50% the number of tertiary care facilities that have emergency-care planning guidelines for children with special health care needs (CSHCN).	23%
J. Integrate pediatric components into the development of all trauma systems	1. Increase to 90% the number of states that fully integrate pediatric elements throughout their state trauma systems.	Triage designations: 24 states and DC

continued

Table 38. (continued)

Goal	Objectives	Baseline
	2. Increase to 85% the number of trauma and tertiary care centers that include rehabilitation professionals as part of the trauma/medical team for pediatric patients during the acute-care phase.	46%
	3. Increase to 35% the number of hospitals that provide or arrange follow-up mental-health services for children and adolescents treated for self-destructive behavior.	2% 7 agencies
K. Ensure a coordi-nated approach to EMS-C	1. Increase by 4 the linkages between key federal agencies and EMS-C-related programs to improve federal coordination of EMS-C issues.	Created in 1995
	2. Create an EMS-C Resource Network Advisory Board that will provide expert advice to the EMS-C program.	10 states
	3. Increase to 50 the number of states participating in annual regional meetings for the promotion of interstate collaboration.	
L. Institutionalize EMS-C within the state EMS system	1. Increase to 56 the number of states and US territories that have developed a specific mechanism for pediatric input into the EMS lead agency.	47 states, 3 US territories and DC
	2. Increase by 5 the number of states that address pediatric issues in state disaster response plans.	0 states

continued

Table 38. *(continued)*

Goal	Objectives	Baseline
M. Improve data-collection systems, data-analysis methodology, and research to describe and evaluate emergency medical care for children	1. Increase to 25 the number of states that produce reports on pediatric issues using their statewide EMS data collection system.	9 states
	2. Increase by 5 the number of cost-benefit analyses completed on pediatric emergency medical services issues.	5 analyses
	3. Increase availability of information related to the effect of managed care on pediatric emergency medical services.	Parent brochure published
	4. Increase by 50% the number of published research papers on EMS-C-related topics.	7 research projects funded
	5. Increase by 50% the number of states that mandate E-coding for injury-related hospitalizations.	17 states

EMS-C Grant Program

The EMS-C program awards several types of grants. The majority are made to states to improve the way in which children receive emergency services. The program also supports grants to enhance knowledge and to develop specialized materials and products, as described in the following paragraphs of this section.

State Grants

State-based grants are of three types: (1) planning grants are designed to enable states that have never had an EMS-C grant to assess needs and do preliminary planning to improve services; (2) implementation grants use existing models of service delivery and system development to implement what is known to improve care; (3) partnership grants provide support to states to continue to improve children's emergency services.

State grantees use their funds for a variety of activities. A few examples follow:

Alaska. The Alaska EMS-C project conducted 19 separate injury-prevention projects. Some targeted large cities and others targeted small rural villages. Efforts included the promotion of bicycle, snowmobile, and all-terrain vehicle safety, water safety, firearm safety, seat-belt usage, installation of smoke detectors, and accessing the emergency medical services system. Recently, a broad-based effort to prevent youth suicide was initiated.

California. The California EMS-C project developed a comprehensive plan for statewide integration of all components of EMS-C into the EMS system and presented it at a state conference to promote its implementation. The state subsequently undertook an evaluation of the plan's implementation.

Maryland. This project coordinated a detailed analysis of ambulance run sheets, which resulted in a recognition of the need for increased training of out-of-hospital personnel in two specific areas: pediatric airway management and the immobilization of cervical spines. The project collaborated with Johns Hopkins University to develop a pediatric airway management course and educational videotape for paramedics. More recent efforts have turned to mass education in pediatric cardiopulmonary resuscitation (CPR) and in the proper use of child safety seats.

New Hampshire. The project developed and promoted a model hospital discharge plan to support families of children with newly acquired disabilities with information and referrals. Special emphasis was placed on the needs of children suffering from traumatic brain injury.

New Mexico. The New Mexico EMS-C project convened a firearm safety task force that included pediatricians, family practitioners, emergency medical technicians (EMTs), firearm enthusiasts, and others. The task force initiated a statewide media campaign—including posters, handbills, and public service announcements—to promote the safe storage of firearms.

New York. The EMS-C project established guidelines for categorization of hospitals for pediatric emergencies, offered training to out-of-hospital and hospital personnel, and conducted research in equipment, triage, treatment, and transport.

North Carolina. North Carolina developed an office emergency preparedness course to assist primary-care and family physicians in taking care of children in emergency situations. The program addresses office equipment and supplies as well as essential assessment and treatment skills. This state has also been instrumental in developing and implementing the Risk-Watch (K-8) childhood injury-prevention curriculum.

Rhode Island. This project developed pediatric-specific protocols for out-of-hospital care. The protocols were integrated into Rhode Island's general EMS protocols. A new "Pedi-Stat" program uses the EMS dispatch system to assist families of children with special healthcare needs in emergency situations through prompt transfer of critical patient information to healthcare physicians.

Targeted-Issue Grants

Targeted-issue grants are intended to support specific, focused activities related to the development of EMS-C capacity, with the intent of providing potential national models.

Examples of targeted-issue grants are:

Connecticut. Through the University of Connecticut Health Center, a new course designed to assist school nurses in managing emergencies more competently was developed.

Missouri. A program called "psychological first aid" was developed at the Children's Mercy Hospital, University of Missouri at Kansas City, to reduce the emotional toll on children ages 5–11 who witness violence. The information on community response to this project was widely disseminated.

New York. The New York University School of Medicine developed a teaching resource for instructors of EMTs. This resource was distributed through CD-ROM, is available on the Internet, and will soon be available on paper. It is designed to assist these instructors in teaching the new emergency medical technician-basic (EMT-B) curriculum.

Oklahoma. Oklahoma has established a training program for child care physicians in childhood injury prevention, first aid, and CPR.

Texas. Through Dallas Children's Hospital, Southwestern Medical Center of Dallas, a project was undertaken to develop a Committee on Pediatric Emergency Medicine in all states, in collaboration with the AAP. Another project in this state is evaluating preparedness of office-based primary-care physicians for handling children needing emergency treatment.

Utah. Utah worked to improve the quality of out-of-hospital emergency care delivered to children who depend on medical technology through notification, training, and model protocols and to develop a database program to prospectively track EMS utilization and link technology-assisted children with EMS runs.

Washington. Washington established community-based drowning-prevention programs throughout the state and integrated drowning prevention into the state EMS/trauma system.

Wisconsin. Wisconsin launched a model childhood poisoning-prevention campaign and has made its campaign materials available for use by other states.

Research Grants

The EMS-C program has also supported a number of research projects, several in collaboration with other agencies. Examples are as follows:

- "Predicting the Need for Hospitalization in Childhood Asthma," Marc Gorelick, University of Pennsylvania.
- "Quality and Cost Containment in Pediatric Intensive Care," John Tilford, Arkansas Children's Hospital.

- "Out-of-Hospital Pediatric Intubation and Patient Outcome," Marianne Gausche, Harbor-UCLA Medical Center.
- "Applying Biomechanical Epidemiology to Injury Prediction," Flaura Winston, Children's Hospital of Philadelphia.
- "Epidemiology and Cost of Emergency Medical Services Provided to Children," Anthony J. Suruda, Rocky Mountain Center for Occupational and Environmental Health.
- "Effectiveness of Regional Trauma Care for Children," Dennis Durbin, University of Pennsylvania.

EMS-C Resource Center and Clearinghouse

EMS-C technical assistance and resource centers have been funded since 1991. These centers help grantees develop new programs, disseminate the products of the EMS-C program, promote public understanding of pediatric concerns in the EMS system, and work with professional organizations to further training efforts in pediatric emergency care for all healthcare professionals.

In fiscal year 1997, a contract was awarded to Children's National Medical Center in Washington, DC, to serve as the EMS-C program's resource center and clearinghouse through fiscal year 2002. It can be reached as follows:

EMS-C National Resource Center
Children's Hospital
111 Michigan Avenue, NW
Washington, DC 20010
Telephone: (202) 884-4927
Web site: http://www.ems-c.org

A second resource center, the National EMS-C Data Analysis Resource Center (NEDARC), provides technical support to the EMS-C community in linking various data sets to improve understanding of the unique needs of children and awareness of areas requiring additional system development.

Programmatic Initiatives

In addition to supporting grants and resource centers, the EMS-C program develops special-topic initiatives, based on emerging concerns or areas where there are clear omissions. Examples of some recent special initiatives follow.

Managed Care and EMS-C

Many efforts have been made to successfully decrease the inappropriate use of emergency services while promoting the concept of accessible quality primary care. Creative managed-care arrangements offer opportunities for some groups to receive primary care that may not have had access to it in the past. However, it is equally important that a quality emergency system be available and that efforts directed at reducing inappropriate use of emergency care not lead to restrictions in appropriate and necessary use.

The EMS-C program's managed-care initiative consists of the following elements:

- White paper series on EMS-C and managed care
- Specialty publications: brochures
- Development of an EMS-C model
- Targeted-issue grants

White Paper Series on EMS-C and Managed Care

The EMS-C program is developing a series of "white papers" to address special topics on the implications of managed care for children's emergency services. Managed-care organizations (MCOs), state and local governments, other purchasers of care, and EMS-C grantees may use the white papers in planning, assessing quality, and initiating children's emergency medical services. To date, very little has been published that addresses pediatric emergency services in a managed-care environment, so the papers will serve an important need. Ten topics have been selected for these papers: (1) 24-hour access to emergency care; (2) access to emergency response systems (ie, 911); (3) quality and accountability for children's EMS; (4) reimbursement for emergency care; (5) definitions of pediatric emergency care; (6) effect of Medicaid managed care on EMS-C; (7) pediatric practice guidelines for EMS; (8) continuity between primary-care physicians and the EMS system; (9) access to pediatric subspecialty care; and (10) injury prevention in managed care. The papers will be published individually, as they become available, and as a compendium when all are completed.

Brochures on EMS-C and Managed Care

One brochure for consumers (parents) has been published and another is planned for purchasers. These brochures raise questions and concerns that parents and purchasers should consider when selecting a managed-care plan.

An EMS-C Model

The EMS-C program is developing a model for the delivery of emergency medical services for children in a managed-care organization. The model will be used to assist state EMS-C leaders, purchasers of care, and others in designing and evaluating managed-care plans. The first step will be a written description that focuses on the entire EMS-C continuum (from injury prevention through rehabilitation). This model will incorporate essential components of EMS-C and will address mechanisms for continuous quality improvement.

Targeted-Issue Grant

A grant was awarded in fiscal year 1997 to the George Washington University to more clearly define the parameters of appropriate EMS-C enrolled in MCOs. It will assess pediatric emergency department use to determine the relationship between perceived and actual need for emergency department services and to identify patterns of payment for emergency department services. Products that will be developed from this grant include:

- An analysis of managed-care contracts and the definition and use of emergency medical services from a legal perspective
- A report on pediatric use of emergency department services and payment patterns
- A model for assessing appropriate use of emergency department services for children in managed care

Poison-Control Initiative

From 1995 to 1999, the EMS-C program has worked to help stabilize the US poison-control center network. These activities were developed in response to the funding crisis facing these centers. Elements of this initiative follow.

Support of Special Studies

The EMS-C program funded an economic analysis of poison-control centers that led to a publication in a peer-review journal identifying the savings that accrue from the presence of a poison-control center. The program also supported an analysis of funding options for both federal and state governments. Another study examined different configurations of poison-control centers and the possible economies of scale related to each. The initial phase of this study was supported by the EMS-C program, and the final phase was supported by the Robert Wood Johnson Foundation. The EMS-C program, through its NEDARC, is linking data sets in Utah to assess the effect of diversion of callers from a 911 dispatcher to the poison-control center. This study should be completed in 1999.

Support of Policy Documents

In collaboration with the Centers for Disease Control and Prevention, the EMS-C program supported a special group (the Poison Control Centers Leadership Group) in the development of a plan for addressing funding problems and other needs of poison-control centers. The plan was submitted to the Department of Health and Human Services Secretary, Donna Shalala, for her consideration in 1997.

Support of Poison-Prevention Activities

The EMS-C program funded a grant in fiscal year 1996 in Wisconsin for the development of materials related to informing the public of steps to take to prevent poisonings. In addition, in fiscal year 1998, the EMS-C program contracted with the American Association of Poison Control Centers to further develop educational materials that can be used by all poison-control centers.

Fostering Collaborative Working Relations: The EMS-C Partnership for Children

The EMS-C program works to better integrate pediatric emergency concerns throughout the continuum of care. In fiscal year 1997, a new initiative was undertaken designed to increase the information about EMS-C available to practitioners from their own associations, to encourage more attention to these concerns, and to foster cross-disciplinary activities. Contracts were developed with 14 professional associations, including the AAP, with each contract including activities related to information dissemination and collaboration. In addition, each contract specifies tasks and objectives in the EMS-C Five Year Plan. Referred to as the EMS Partnership for Children, the group meets twice yearly to share information and experiences. The EMS-C program also developed a special project in collaboration with the American Academy of Pediatrics and the American College of Emergency Physicians in 1997. Called the EMS-C Coordinating Committee, this group develops joint projects and policies, enabling the physician community to "speak with one voice" on pediatric emergency-care issues.

Other Special Initiatives

The EMS-C program has undertaken other special initiatives in the past few years, in addition to those heretofore described. For example, through the National EMS-C Resource Alliance, national consensus documents were developed on pediatric equipment for transport vehicles and on pediatric equipment for hospital emergency departments, as well as a research agenda for EMS-C. These documents were published simultaneously in three journals. Other examples of topics on which considerable work has been done include: children and disasters; children with special health care needs; family-centered care in emergencies; cultural competence; injury prevention; data collection and analysis; and public relations for EMS-C.

Resources and Information on the EMS-C Grant Program

Grant priorities for the EMS-C program are announced annually, typically in late winter or early spring, and at that time application kits become available. The program's authorizing legislation limits eligibility for EMS-C grants either to states or to schools of medicine. Application kits may be obtained by telephoning the HRSA Grants Application Center at (888) 333-4772.

Updated information on the EMS-C program, including grant program guidance, is also available on the EMS-C Web site: http://www.ems-c.org.

For additional information on the EMS-C program, contact:

Cindy Doyle, RN or
David Heppel, MD
Maternal and Child Health
  Bureau
Room 18-A-39
5600 Fishers Lane
Rockville, MD 20857
Telephone: (301) 443-2250

Jeff Michael, PhD, or
Garry Criddle, RN
National Highway Traffic
  Safety Administration
NTS-42
400 7th Street, SW
Washington, DC 20590
Telephone: (202) 366-5440

Suggested Reading

Emergency Medical Services for Children National Resource Center. *Five Year Plan, Midcourse Review: Emergency Medical Services for Children, 1995–2000.* Washington, DC: Maternal and Child Health Bureau, Health Resources and Services Administration, and National Highway Traffic Safety Administration, Department of Transportation; 1997

Feely, HB, Athey, JL. EMSC: *Emergency Medical Services for Children: 10 Year Report.* Arlington, VA: National Center for Education in Maternal and Child Health; 1995

Henderson DP. The Los Angeles pediatric emergency care system. *J Emerg Nurs.* 1988;14:96–100

Institute of Medicine, Committee on Pediatric Emergency Medical Services. Durch JS, Lohr KN, eds. *Emergency Medical Services for Children.* Washington, DC: National Academy Press; 1993

Ramenofsky ML, Luterman A, Quindlen E, Riddick L, Curreri PW. Maximum survival in pediatric trauma: the ideal system. *J Trauma.* 1984;24:818–823

Seidel JS, Hornbein M, Yoshiyama K, Kuznets D, Finklestein JZ, St. Geme JW Jr. Emergency medical services and the pediatric patient: are the needs being met? *Pediatrics.* 1984;73;769–772

US Department of Health and Human Services, Health Resources and Services Administration, Maternal and Child Health Bureau. *Emergency Medical Services for Children: Abstracts of Active Projects Fiscal Year 1997.* Torrance, CA: National Emergency Medical Services for Children Resource Alliance; 1997

Glossary

AAP American Academy of Pediatrics. A professional organization of board-certified pediatricians and others who care for children in their practices.

ACEP American College of Emergency Physicians. A professional organization of board-certified emergency medicine physicians.

ACS American College of Surgeons. A professional organization of board-certified surgeons.

AHA American Heart Association. A professional organization dedicated to the prevention of heart disease and stroke.

APLS Advanced Pediatric Life Support. A course developed by the AAP and ACEP that concentrates on education in pediatric emergency medicine.

ATLS Advanced Trauma Life Support. A course developed by the American College of Surgeons and targeted to those who provide advanced trauma life support.

BLS Basic Life Support. A course developed by the AHA to provide basic life-support skills.

BTLS Basic Trauma Life Support. A course designed to teach the basics of the initial resuscitation of the trauma patient.

CAAMS Commission on the Accreditation of Air Medical Services.

CAMTS Commission on the Accreditation of Air Medical Transport Services.

CAPTA Child Abuse Prevention and Treatment Act. A statute governing child-abuse-reporting requirements.

COPEM Committee on Pediatric Emergency Medicine. An official AAP committee that works on matters related to access to and delivery of pediatric emergency care.

CPS Child Protective Services. A social service agency that has jurisdiction for child protection.

CS Conscious sedation. A medically controlled state of depressed consciousness that allows protective reflexes to be maintained; retains the patient's ability to maintain a patent airway, independently and continuously; and permits appropriate response by the patient to physical stimulation and verbal command.

CSHCN Children with Special Health Care Needs. Children who have or who are at increased risk for a chronic physical, developmental, behavioral, or emotional condition and who require help and related services of a type or amount beyond that required by children generally.

DS Deep Sedation. Level of depressed consciousness or unconsciousness from which the patient is not easily aroused and does not respond purposefully to physical stimulation or verbal command.

ED Emergency Department.

EDAP Emergency Department Approved for Pediatrics. An ED that has demonstrated a commitment to pediatric emergency care by meeting guidelines for staffing, equipment, and supplies, as well as continuous quality improvement (CQI) and other policies and procedures specifically related to pediatric patents.

EIF Emergency Information Form. An information sheet that contains data about the health status of children with special health care needs.

EMS Emergency Medical Services. A system of emergency care that is usually administered by the government and that provides out-of-hospital care.

EMS-C Emergency Medical Services for Children. A comprehensive system of services integrated into existing community and EMS resources.

EMT Emergency medical technician.

EMTALA Emergency Medical Treatment and Labor Act. A federal statute that covers requirements for emergency treatment.

ENA Emergency Nurses Association. A professional organization of nurses who work in emergency medicine.

ENPC Emergency Nursing Pediatric Course. A course developed and given by the Emergency Nurses Association.

HRSA Health Resources and Services Administration.

IEMP Individual Emergency Medical Plan. A plan developed for children with special healthcare needs.

ISP Internet Service Provider. Serves as a middleman between the computer user and the Internet providing the physical connection to the Internet.

MCHB Maternal and Child Health Bureau. A division of the US Department of Health and Human Services.

MCO Managed-care organization.

MSE Medical Screening Examination. An examination that is required under the EMTALA to determine if emergency care must be rendered.

NASN National Association of School Nurses.

NASSNC National Association of School Nurse Consultants.

NEDARC National EMS-C Data Analysis Resource Center. A national EMS-C center located at the University of Utah and funded to assist EMS-C projects with data collection and analysis.

NERA The National EMS-C Resource Center. A center for research and product development for the emergency care of children, located on the campus of Harbor-UCLA Medical Center in Torrance, CA.

NHTSA The National Highway Traffic Safety Administration. A division of the US Department of Transportation.

NRC The National EMS-C Resource Center. Serves as a US resource center for all federal EMS-C activities.

NRP Neonatal Resuscitation Program. An educational program sponsored by the AAP and AHA to teach newborn resuscitation and administered by the AAP.

PACU Pediatric Acute Care Unit.

PALS Pediatric Advanced Life Support. A course, offered by the AHA and AAP, that concentrates on cardiopulmonary resuscitation and training.

PBLS Pediatric Basic Life Support. A course in basic pediatric life support sponsored by the AAP and AHA and administered through the AHA.

PCCC Pediatric Critical Care Center. A pediatric referral center that provides tertiary services to critically ill and injured children.

PEM Pediatric Emergency Medicine. A subboarded specialty within Pediatrics and Emergency Medicine.

PFA Psychological First Aid. An approach to the care of the child who has witnessed violence.

PICU Pediatric Intensive Care Unit. An intensive care unit designed and staffed to care for critically ill and injured children.

PRISM Pediatric Risk of Mortality Score. A score used by pediatric intensivists to measure the risk of mortality of patients admitted to the PICU. The score is often used to compare risk and outcome to determine the quality of care offered to patients.

Prudent Layperson Definition of an Emergency In statute: If a patient presents with symptoms that a "prudent layperson" could reasonably expect to impair one's health, then it is to be considered an emergency for reimbursement purposes.

PTC Pediatric Trauma Center. A trauma center that meets state or ACS criteria or both to manage the acutely traumatized child.

RSI Rapid sequence intubation. The use of medications to facilitate the rapid endotracheal intubation of an adult or child.

SCCM Society for Critical Care Medicine.

SNEMS-C School Nurses EMS-C Program. An educational program developed by the Connecticut EMS-C Program.

WWW World Wide Web.

Resources

National Associations, Organizations, and Resource Centers

AAP Publications Resource List

First Aid/Choking/CPR Chart

National Associations, Organizations, and Resource Centers

American Academy of
  Pediatrics
141 Northwest Point Boulevard
Elk Grove Village, IL 60007
Telephone: (847) 228-5005
(800) 433-9016

American College of Emer-
  gency Physicians
PO Box 619911
Dallas, TX 75261-9911
Telephone: (972) 550-0911
(800) 798-1822

American Heart Association
7272 Greenville Avenue
Dallas, TX 75231
Telephone: (214) 373-6300
(800) AHA-USA1

American Red Cross
431 18th Street, NW
Washington, DC 20006
Telephone: (202) 728-6400

American Trauma Society
8903 Presidential Parkway,
  Suite 512
Upper Marlboro, MD 20772
Telephone: (301) 420-4189
(800) 556-7890

Children's Safety Network
1400 Eye Street, NW, Suite 200
Washington, DC 20005
Telephone: (202) 842-4450

Citizen CPR Foundation
c/o Ms Mary Newman
PO Box 911
Carmel, IN 46032
Telephone: (317) 843-1940

EMSC National Resource Center
111 Michigan Avenue, NW
Washington, DC 20010
Telephone: (202) 884-4927

Emergency Nurses
  Association
216 Higgins Road
Park Ridge, IL 60068
Telephone: (847) 460-4000
(800) 900-9659

International Association of
  Fire Fighters
1750 New York Avenue, NW
Washington, DC 20006
Telephone: (202) 737-8484

Medic Alert Foundation,
  International
2323 Colorado Avenue
Turlock, CA 95382
Telephone: (209) 668-3333

National Association of EMS
  Physicians
PO Box 15945-281
Lenexa, KS 66285-5945
Telephone: (913) 492-5858
(800) 228-3677

National Association of EMTs
102 West Leake Street
Clinton, MS 39056
Telephone: (601) 924-7744
(800) 346-2368

National Association of State
  EMS Directors
111 Park Place
Falls Church, VA 22046
Telephone: (703) 538-1799

National EMS Alliance
408 Monroe Street
Clinton, MS 39056
Telephone: (601) 924-3235

National EMSC Data Analysis
  Resource Center
410 Chipeta Way, Suite 222
Salt Lake City, UT 84108
Telephone: (801) 581-6410

National Emergency Number
  Association
47849 Paper Mill Road
Coshocton, OH 43812-9724
Telephone: (800) 332-3911

National Rural Health
  Association
One West Armour Boulevard,
  Suite 301
Kansas City, MO 64111
Telephone: (816) 756-3140

National Safe Kids Campaign
1301 Pennsylvania Avenue, NW
  Suite 100
Washington, DC 20004-1707
Telephone: (202) 662-0600

National Safety Council
1121 Spring Lake Drive
Itasca, IL 60143
Telephone: (630) 285-1121
(800) 621-7619

Government Agencies

Centers for Disease Control
  and Prevention
National Center for Injury
  Prevention and Control
1600 Clifton Road, NE,
  Mailstop F-36
Atlanta, GA 30333
Telephone: (404) 639-3311
(800) 311-3435

Federal Interagency Committee
  on EMS
US Fire Administration
Federal Emergency Manage-
  ment Agency
16825 South Seton Avenue
Emmitsburg, MD 21727
Telephone: (301) 447-1080
(800) 238-3358

US Department of Health and Human Services
Maternal and Child Health Bureau
5600 Fishers Lane, Room 18-A-30
Rockville, MD 20857
Telephone: (301) 443-2250
(800) 688-9889

US Department of Transportation
National Highway Traffic Safety Administration
400 Seventh Street, SW
Washington, DC 20590-0001
Telephone: (202) 366-5440
(800) 424-9393

AAP Publications Resource List

For Parents

Brochures

Alcohol: Your Child and Drugs
Allergies in Children
Bronchiolitis and Your Young Child
Child Care
Child Sexual Abuse: What It Is and How to Prevent It
Choking Prevention and First Aid for Infants and Children
Cocaine: Your Child and Drugs
Croup and Your Young Child
Diarrhea and Dehydration
Ear Infections and Children
Family Shopping Guide to Car Seats
Febrile Seizures
Guide to Children's Dental Health
Guide to Children's Medications
How to Help Your Child With Asthma
Immunizations: What You Need to Know
Infant Sleep Positioning and SIDS
Inhalant Abuse: Your Child and Drugs
Keep Your Family Safe From Firearm Injury
Marijuana: Your Child and Drugs
Middle Ear Fluid in Young Children
Minor Head Injuries in Children
Parent's Guide to Water Safety
Playground Safety
Protect Your Child From Poison
Raising Children to Resist Violence
Surviving: Coping With Adolescent Depression and Suicide
The Teen Driver
Toy Safety
Your Child and Antibiotics
Your Child and the Environment

Fact Sheets and Forms

Air Bag Safety Facts
Baby Walkers Are Very Dangerous

Emergency Information Form for Children With Special Health
  Care Needs
Home Safety Checklist
Infant Sleep Positioning and SIDS
One-Minute Car Seat Safety Check-Up
Trampolines
When Your Child Needs Emergency Medical Services Fact Sheet

First Aid/Choking/CPR Chart

Life Support Course
Pediatric Basic Life Support (cosponsored with and available
  through the American Heart Association)

Parenting Books
Caring for Your Baby and Young Child: Birth to Age 5
Caring for Your School-Age Child: Ages 5 to 12
Caring for Your Adolescent: Ages 12 to 21
Guide to Your Child's Nutrition
Guide to Your Child's Sleep
Guide to Your Child's Symptoms
Your Baby's First Year

TIPP Safety Slips
About Bicycle Helmets
Baby-Sitting Reminders
Bicycle Safety: Myths and Facts
Child as Passenger on an Adult's Bicycle
Choosing the Right Size Bicycle for Your Child
Home Water Hazards for Young Children
Infant Furniture: Cribs
Lawn Mower Safety
Life Jackets and Life Preservers
Pool Safety for Children
Protect Your Child...Prevent Poisoning
Protect Your Home Against Fire
Safe Bicycling Starts Early
Safety Tips for Home Playground Equipment
Safe Driving: A Parental Responsibility
Tips for Getting Your Kids to Wear Helmets
Water Safety for Your School-Age Child

Videos

Caring for Your Newborn: A Parent's Guide to the First 3 Months
Fit for a King: The Smart Kid's Guide to Food and Fun
Mastering Asthma: A Family Guide
Your Child's Anesthesia

For Health Professionals

Broselow™ Pediatric Emergency Tape

Life Support Programs

APLS: The Pediatric Emergency Medicine Course
Neonatal Resuscitation Program
Pediatric Advanced Life Support (cosponsored with and available
  through the American Heart Association)
Pediatric Education for Prehospital Professionals Course

Manuals and Handbooks for Health Professionals

Anesthesia and Pain Management for the Pediatrician
Coding for Pediatrics
Drugs for Pediatric Emergencies
Guidelines for Air and Ground Transport of Neonatal and Pediatric Patients
Guidelines for Health Supervision
Handbook of Common Poisonings in Children
Health in Day Care
Injury Prevention and Control for Children and Youth
Pediatric Dosage Handbook
Pediatric Environmental Health
Pediatric Nutrition Handbook
Pediatric Telephone Protocols
Red Book: Report of the Committee on Infectious Diseases
School Health: Policy and Practice

Model Bills

All-Terrain Vehicle Regulation Act
Child Abuse Victim Protection Act
Child Bicycle Safety Act
Child Death Investigation Act

Child Health Insurance Reform Plan (CHIRP)
Childhood Vaccine Act
Graduated Drivers' Licensing Act
Medicaid Principles and Sample Legislative Language
Medical Liability Statute of Limitations Reform Act
Newborn Health Insurance Law
Pediatric Emergency Medical Services Act
Personal Flotation Device Act
Post-Delivery Care for Mothers and Newborns Act
Protection of Children From Handguns Act
Swimming Pool Safety Act
Vaccine Injury Act
Vehicle Operator Permit Delay and Suspension Act

Policy Statements Related to EMSC

Committee on Pediatric Emergency Medicine
Access to Emergency Medical Care
Consensus Report for Regionalization of Services for
  Critically Ill or Injured Children
Consent for Medical Services for Children and
  Adolescents
Death of a Child in the Emergency Department
Emergency Physician and the Office-Based Pediatrician:
  An EMSC Team
Guidelines for Pediatric Emergency Care Facilities
Pediatrician's Role in Advocating Life Support Courses
  for Parents
Pediatrician's Role in Disaster Preparedness
Recommendations for Freestanding Urgent Care Facilities
Role of the Pediatrician in Rural EMSC
Use of Physical Restraint Interventions for Children and
  Adolescents in the Acute Care Setting

Committee on Adolescence
Firearms and Adolescents
Sexual Assault and the Adolescent
Suicide and Suicide Attempts in Adolescents and Young Adults

Transition of Care Provided for Adolescents With Special
Health Care Needs

Committee on Bioethics
Ethics and the Care of Critically Ill Infants and Children
Guidelines on Forgoing Life Sustaining Medical Treatment
Informed Consent, Parental Permission, and Assent in
Pediatric Practice
Religious Objections to Medical Care

Committee on Child Abuse and Neglect
Distinguishing Sudden Infant Death Syndrome From Child
Abuse Fatalities
Guidelines for the Evaluation of Sexual Abuse of Children
Investigation and Review of Unexpected Infant and Child Deaths
Oral and Dental Aspects of Child Abuse and Neglect
Public Disclosure of Private Information About Victims
of Abuse
Role of the Pediatrician in Recognizing and Intervening
on Behalf of Abused Women
Shaken Baby Syndrome: Inflicted Cerebral Trauma

Committee on Child Health Financing
Guiding Principles for Managed Care Arrangements for the
Health Care of Infants, Adolescents, and Young Adults

Committee on Community Health Services
Health Needs of Homeless Children and Families
Health Care for Children of Farm Worker Families
Health Care for Children of Immigrant Families

Committee on Drugs
Alternative Routes of Drug Administration–Advantages and
Disadvantages
Drugs for Pediatric Emergencies

Committee on Hospital Care
Facilities and Equipment for the Care of Pediatric Patients in
a Community Hospital
Guidelines for Developing Admission and Discharge Policies
for the PICU
Guidelines and Levels of Care for Pediatric Intensive Care Units

Physician's Role in Coordinating Care of Hospitalized Children
Medical Necessity for Hospitalization of the Abused **and** Neglected Child
Precertification Process

Committee on Injury and Poison Prevention
All-Terrain Vehicles
Bicycle Helmets
Children and Fireworks
Children in Pickup Trucks
Drowning in Infants, Children, and Adolescents
Efforts to Reduce the Toll of Injuries in Childhood Require Expanded Research
55 Miles Per Hour Maximum Speed Limit
Firearm Injuries Affecting the Pediatric Population
Hospital Discharge Data on Injury: The Need for E Codes
Injuries Associated With Infant Walkers
Injuries Related to "Toy" Firearms
In-Line Skating Injuries in Children and Adolescents
Office-Based Counseling for Injury Prevention
Prevention of Unintentional Injury Among American Indian and Alaska Native Children
Ride-On Mower Injuries in Children
Rural Injuries
Safe Transportation of Newborns Discharged From the Hospital
Safe Transportation of Premature and Low Birth Weight Infants
School Bus Transportation of Children With Special Needs
School Transportation Safety
Selecting and Using the Most Appropriate Car Safety Seats for Growing Children
Skateboard Injuries
Snowmobile Statement
Teenage Driver
Trampolines at Home, School, and Recreational Centers
Transporting Children With Special Needs

Committee on Psychosocial Aspects of Child and Family Health
How Pediatricians Can Respond to the Psychosocial Implications of Disasters
Pediatricians and Childhood Bereavement

Committee on School Health
Basic Life Support Training in School
Guidelines for Urgent Care in School

Committee on Sports Medicine
Cardiac Dysrhythmias and Sports
Climatic Heat Stress and the Exercising Child
Exercise and the Asthmatic Child
Horseback Riding and Head Injuries
Infant Swimming Programs
Mitral Valve Prolapse and Athletic Participation in Children and Adolescents

Section on Anesthesiology
Evaluation and Preparation of Pediatric Patients Undergoing Anesthesia
Guidelines for the Pediatric Perioperative Anesthesia Environment

Task Force on Adolescent Assault Victim Needs
Adolescent Assault Victim Needs: A Review of Issues and a Model Protocol

Task Force on Medical Informatics
Safeguards Needed in the Transfer of Patient Data

Task Force on Violence
Role of the Pediatrician in Youth Violence Prevention

Practice Parameters
Management of Acute Gastroenteritis in Young Children
Management of Hyperbilirubinemia in the Healthy Term Newborn
Management of Minor Closed Head Injury
Managing Otitis Media with Effusion in Young Children
The Neurodiagnostic Evaluation of the Child with a First Simple Febrile Seizure

Speaker/Slide Kits
Emergency Medical Services for Children: A Child's Life Depends
  On It
Visual Diagnosis of Child Physical Abuse
Visual Diagnosis of Child Sexual Abuse

TIPP–The Injury Prevention Program
Age-Related Safety Sheets
Parent Counseling Sheets
Safety Surveys

Vaccine Information Sheets

Videos/CD-ROM
Focus on Child Abuse: Resources for Prevention, Recognition,
  and Treatment (CD)
Intubating the Newborn (video)
PediaStat: For Pediatric Urgent Care and Emergency Medicine (CD)
Safe Active Play: A Guide to Avoiding Play Area Hazards (video)

To order materials contact:

American Academy of Pediatrics
PO Box 747
Elk Grove Village, IL 60009-0747
(888) 227-1770 or (847) 228-5005
Fax: (847) 228-1281
http://www.aap.org

FIRST AID

Call 911 or an Emergency Number for any severely ill or injured child.

EYE INJURIES

If anything is splashed in the eye, flush gently with water for at least 15 minutes. Call the Poison Center or your doctor for further advice. Any injured or painful eye should be seen by a doctor. Do **NOT** touch or rub an injured eye. Do **NOT** apply medication. Do **NOT** remove objects stuck into the eye. Cover the painful or injured eye with a paper cup or eye shield until you can get medical help.

FRACTURES AND SPRAINS

DO NOT MOVE A CHILD WHO MAY HAVE A NECK OR BACK INJURY, as this may cause serious harm. Call 911 or an emergency number.

If an injured area is painful, swollen, deformed, or if motion causes pain, wrap it in a towel or soft cloth and make a splint to immobilize the arm or leg with cardboard or another rigid material. Apply ice or a cold compress, call your doctor, or seek emergency care. If there is a break in the skin near the fracture, or if you can see the bone, cover the area with a clean dressing and make a splint as described above.

If the foot or hand below the injured part is cold or discolored, seek immediate emergency care.

HEAD INJURIES

DO NOT MOVE A CHILD WHO MAY HAVE A SERIOUS HEAD AND/OR NECK OR BACK INJURY. This may cause further harm.

Call 911 or an emergency number for a child with a head injury and any of the following:

■ Any loss of consciousness or drowsiness
■ Persistent headache or vomiting
■ Clumsiness or inability to move any body part
■ Oozing of blood or watery fluid from ears or nose
■ Convulsions (Seizures)
■ Abnormal speech or behavior

For any questions about less serious injuries, call your doctor.

BURNS AND SCALDS

General Treatment First stop the burning process by removing the child from contact with hot water or a hot object (eg, tar). If clothing is burning, do not remove. Smother the flames and wet the clothes immediately in order to stop further burning and pain. Run cool water over burned skin until the pain stops. Do not use ice or apply any medication or ointment.

Burns With Blisters Do not break the blisters. Call your doctor for advice on how to cover the burn and about any large burns or burns on the face, hands, feet, or genitals.

Large or Deep Burns Call 911 or an emergency number. After stopping and cooling the burn, keep the child warm with a clean sheet covered with a blanket until help arrives.

Electrical Burns Disconnect electrical power. Do **NOT** touch the victim with bare hands. Pull the victim away from the power source with wood or a thick, dry cloth. **ALL** electrical burns need to be seen by a doctor.

POISONS

If the child has been exposed to or ingested a poison, call your Poison Center.

Swallowed Poisons Any non-food substance is a potential poison. Call the Poison Center immediately. Do not induce vomiting except on professional advice. The Poison Center will give you further instructions.

Fumes, Gases, or Smoke Call 911 or the fire department and get the victim into fresh air. If the child is not breathing, start CPR and continue until help arrives.

NOSEBLEEDS

Keep the child in a sitting position with the head tilted slightly forward. Apply firm steady pressure to both nostrils by squeezing them between your thumb and index finger for 10 minutes. If bleeding continues, or is very heavy, call your doctor or seek emergency care.

STINGS AND BITES

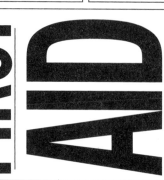

Stinging Insects Remove the stinger as quickly as possible with the scraping motion of a fingernail. Put a cold compress on the bite to relieve the pain. If hives, nausea, vomiting, trouble breathing, or fainting occurs, call your doctor or 911. For spider bites, call your doctor or Poison Center and describe the spider.

Animal or Human Bites Wash wound thoroughly with soap and water. Call your doctor.

Ticks Place tweezers as close as possible to the head of the tick and slowly pull the tick away from the point of attachment. Call your doctor if any parts of the tick remain under the skin or if the child develops symptoms such as a rash or fever.

Snake Bites Keep the child at rest. Call the Poison Center. Do not apply ice. Loosely splint the injured extremity. Take the child to an emergency department. Keep the extremity at rest, positioned at, or slightly below, the level of the heart.

FEVER

Fever in children is usually caused by infection, too warm an environment, or prolonged overactivity. Take the child's temperature to document a fever. The height of fever is less important than the child's appearance and activity. If the child appears very ill with fever, or is less than 3 months old, call your doctor. When the temperature reaches 102°F, undress the child to a diaper or underpants and a t-shirt, give fever medication as recommended by your doctor or the package instructions, and provide plenty of cool liquids to drink.

If the temperature remains over 104°F, sponge your child with lukewarm water (slightly cooler than the child's skin), and call your doctor. Do not use cold water or rubbing alcohol to sponge your child. If you are sponging your child in the tub, do not fill the tub with more than 2 inches of water, and do not leave the child unattended.

TEETH

Baby Teeth If knocked out or broken, apply clean gauze to control bleeding and call your dentist.

Permanent Teeth If knocked out, find the tooth and, if dirty, rinse gently without scrubbing or touching the root. Do not use chemical cleansers. Use milk or cold running water. Place the tooth into clean water or milk and transport the tooth with the child when seeking emergency care. Call and go directly to your dentist or an emergency department. If the tooth is broken, save the pieces in milk and call your dentist immediately.

CONVULSIONS, SEIZURES

Protect the child from injury. Put nothing in the child's mouth. Loosen any restrictive clothing. Perform rescue breathing if the child is blue or not breathing. If breathing, lay the child on his or her side to prevent choking. Call 911 or an emergency number.

SKIN WOUNDS

Make sure your child is immunized for tetanus. Puncture wounds or lacerations may require a tetanus booster even when your child is currently immunized.

Bruises Apply cold compresses. Call your doctor for a crush injury, large bruises, continued pain, or swelling.

Cuts Wash small cuts with water until clean; topical antiseptics can be used. Use direct pressure with a clean cloth to stop bleeding. Apply a topical antibiotic ointment, then cover the cut with clean dressing. Call your doctor for large and deep cuts since stitches should be placed without delay. Apply pressure directly to the wound for major bleeding with a clean cloth and call for help (911). Continue pressure until help arrives.

Scrapes Irrigate with water to remove dirt and germs. Do not use detergents, alcohol, or peroxide. Use a topical antiseptic. Apply an antibiotic ointment and a nonadherent dressing.

Splinters Remove small splinters with tweezers, then wash and apply topical antiseptic. If you are unable to remove the splinter completely, call your doctor.

Puncture Wounds Do not remove large objects such as a knife or stick from a wound. Call for emergency medical assistance (911). Such objects must be removed by a doctor. Call your doctor for all puncture wounds. Your child may need a tetanus booster.

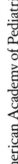

Skin Exposure If acids, lye, pesticides, chemicals, poisonous plants, or any potentially poisonous substance comes in contact with a child's skin, eyes, or hair, brush off any residual material while wearing rubber gloves, if possible. Remove contaminated clothing. Wash skin, eyes, or hair with large quantities of water or mild soap and water. Call the Poison Center for further advice.

If a child is unconscious, becoming drowsy, having convulsions, or having trouble breathing, call 911 or an emergency number. Bring the poisonous substance (safely contained) with you to the hospital.

FAINTING

Lay the child on his or her back with the head to the side. Do **NOT** give the child anything to drink. If the child does not wake up right away, call your doctor, or dial 911 or your emergency number. If the child is not breathing, begin CPR.

Does your community have 911? If not, note the number of your local ambulance service and other important numbers below.

BE PREPARED: CALL 911
KEEP EMERGENCY NUMBERS BY YOUR TELEPHONE

DOCTOR _____

POISON CENTER _____

AMBULANCE _____

EMERGENCY DEPT. _____

FIRE _____

POLICE _____

American Academy of Pediatrics

WARNER LAMBERT Supported by an educational grant from Warner-Lambert

Turn Over for Choking and CPR Instructions

HE0008 (Rev. 1/99)
© American Academy of Pediatrics

CHOKING/CPR

Call 911 or an Emergency Number after starting rescue efforts.
LEARN AND PRACTICE CPR

FOR INFANTS UNDER ONE YEAR

INFANT CHOKING

Begin the following if the infant is choking and is unable to breathe. However, if the infant is coughing, crying, or speaking, DO NOT do any of the following, but call your doctor for further advice.

1 FIVE BACK BLOWS

2 FIVE CHEST THRUSTS

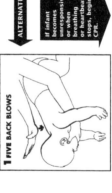

ALTERNATING

If infant becomes unresponsive or when breathing or heartbeat stops, begin CPR.

INFANT CPR
Cardiopulmonary Resuscitation
To be used when infant is unresponsive or when breathing or heartbeat stops.

1 OPEN AIRWAY
- **Look** for movement of the chest and abdomen
- **Listen** for sounds of breathing
- **Feel** for breath on your cheek
- **Open** airway as shown
- **Remove** foreign object if present; sweep it out with finger only if seen

2 RESCUE BREATHING
- **Position** head and chin with both hands as shown
- **Seal** your mouth over mouth and nose
- **Blow gently,** enough air to make chest rise and fall two times

If no rise or fall, repeat 1 & 2. If no response, treat for obstructed airway. (See "INFANT CHOKING" steps 1 & 2 above.)

3 FEEL FOR PULSE AS SHOWN
- **Pulse present,** continue 1 breath every 3 seconds
- **No pulse,** start chest compressions

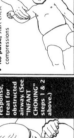

4 CHEST COMPRESSIONS
- **Compress** chest 1/2″ to 1″
- **Alternate** 5 fast compressions with 1 breath
- **Compress** chest 100 times per minute

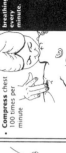

Check for return of pulse and breathing every minute.

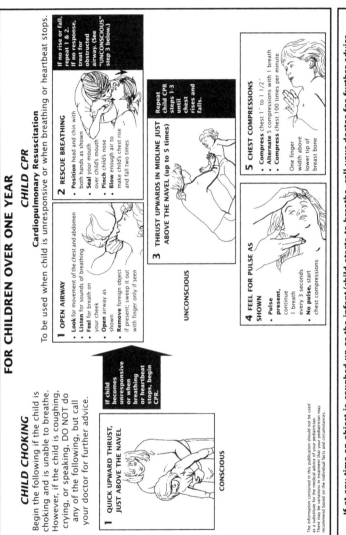

To order copies of this chart, contact:
American Academy of Pediatrics
PO Box 747
Elk Grove Village, IL 60009-0747
(888) 227-1770 or (847) 228-5005
Fax: (847) 228-1281   http://www.aap.org

Index